INTERVENTION STRATEGIES FOR CHANGING HEALTH BEHAVIOR

Changing habits, particularly habits that are self-destructive and unhealthy, is among the most challenging goals of therapists and coaches who work with clients in promoting a healthier lifestyle. The purpose of this book is to "help the helper," that is, to assist the person whose professional mission it is to provide a service that enables clients or patients to acknowledge their unhealthy habits and to replace them with more desirable, healthier routines. It focuses on the power of helping clients identify: (1) the inconsistency between their core values—what they consider most important in life—and one or more unhealthy habits, (2) the costs and long-term consequences of this inconsistency, called a "disconnect" in the model, and (3) their willingness to conclude that the consequences of this inconsistency are unacceptable. At that stage, (4) clients should be prepared to work with a coach in developing and carrying out an action plan that aims to remove the disconnect between the client's values and at least one of the unhealthy habits.

Mark H. Anshel is professor emeritus at Middle Tennessee State University in Murfreesboro, Tennessee. He received a degree in physical education from Illinois State University (B.S.) and degrees from McGill University (M.A.) and Florida State University (Ph.D.) in performance psychology. He has authored over 140 research articles published in scientific journals, 14 book chapters, and 10 books, including *Applied Health Fitness Psychology* (2014). Over the past 15 years, he developed, validated, and authored research articles on the Disconnected Values Model.

INTERVENTION STRATEGIES FOR CHANGING HEALTH BEHAVIOR

Applying the Disconnected Values Model

Mark H. Anshel, Ph.D.

Routledge
Taylor & Francis Group
NEW YORK AND LONDON

First published 2016
by Routledge
605 Third Avenue, New York, NY 10017

and by Routledge
4 Park Square, Milton Park, Abingdon, Oxon OX14 4RN

Routledge is an imprint of the Taylor & Francis Group, an informa business

Library of Congress Cataloging-in-Publication Data

Anshel, Mark H. (Mark Howard), author. Intervention strategies for changing health behavior : applying the disconnected values model / Mark H. Anshel. New York, NY : Psychology Press, 2016. | Includes bibliographical references and index. Counseling—methods. | Health Behavior. | Habits. LCC RC489. B4 | NLM W 85 | DDC 616.89/1—dc23

ISBN: 978-1-138-90811-6 (hbk)
ISBN: 978-1-138-90812-3 (pbk)
ISBN: 978-1-315-65162-0 (ebk)

Typeset in Bembo
by Apex CoVantage, LLC

CONTENTS

PREFACE

The purpose of this book is to "help the helper," that is, to assist the person whose professional mission it is to provide a service that enables clients (or patients) to acknowledge their unhealthy habits and to replace them with more desirable, healthier routines. Health behavior change is the responsibility of educators, medical practitioners, mental health professionals, dieticians, and fitness coaches, as well as others who provide clients with the incentive to lead a more productive and happy life.

Perhaps one of the most perplexing questions about human behavior is why we do things every single day that we know are bad for us. We do not obtain adequate sleep, we often go nonstop all day without taking a recovery break, we hurriedly eat high-fat foods, we feel stressed, and we are controlled by the demands and expectations of others. Are we not aware of these behavioral and emotional tendencies? Do we not realize the health-related consequences of our behavior patterns? Why do we act in ways that are not in our best interests?

The reasons we maintain "bad" habits—why we persist in a self-destructive lifestyle—and make poor choices about unhealthy behavior patterns remain a mystery. How to help someone stop engaging in self-destructive behaviors and to change his or her lifestyle, however, is more challenging because it is deeply embedded in the person's day-to-day schedule and within his or her comfort zone. Changing behavior that influences a person's health is the main focus of this book.

This book is for mental health professionals, fitness coaches, registered dieticians, and anyone else in the industry—professional or student—who tries to improve the health behavior of their clients or patients using a formal intervention called the Disconnected Values Model. It is the *psychology* of health behavior change that has received surprisingly little attention in the education and training of our health care professionals to influence client behavior. This book focuses on providing a novel approach, supported by empirical research, to improve the effectiveness of changing client attitudes, emotions, motivation, and behavior for developing and maintaining a healthy lifestyle.

Although adopted for use in university settings, the primary audience for this book is professionals who are devoted to changing the health behavior of clients and patients and to make a difference in people's lives. The process for health behavior change is called the Disconnected Values Model (DVM), which consists of a series of stages that has shown to be effective for helping people replace unhealthy habits with new, healthier ones. While removing a habit is a very challenging task for any health professional, especially when it comes to increasing physical activity and changing eating patterns, perhaps we can mobilize a group of motivated and informed professionals to change a culture that promotes sedentary behavior and overeating. Lifestyle change cannot be forced, but by juxtaposing the benefits of a healthier lifestyle with the many short-term costs and long-term consequences of a sedentary lifestyle and linking people to a vast network of social support such as health professionals, fitness leaders, and registered dieticians, we can slowly begin the process of changing the way we live.

The key issue to using the DVM is to follow the predetermined sequence of activities—the DVM's components—that performs four main functions: (1) to help clients acknowledge one or more unhealthy habits, (2) to determine that each unhealthy habit has benefits (or else we would not continue the habit, however bad for us) and consequences, (3) to identify our most important values, some of which are inconsistent with one or more unhealthy habits, and (4) to conclude that the consequences of this "disconnect" between habits and values is unacceptable. This is the heart of the DVM because if a client makes this conclusion, he or she is ready to work with health professionals to generate and carry out an action plan. The plan's aim is to remove the disconnect and facilitate the consistency between the client's values and unhealthy habits. The DVM has been shown to be a highly effective intervention to change health-related behavior and selected emotions, attitudes, and mental health in numerous published studies in reputable scientific journals. Some of these studies are reviewed in the book.

This 20-chapter book is divided into four parts. Part 1 (chapters 1–2) consists of various explanations of our self-destructive nature, that is, why we maintain habits that we—individually and culturally—know are unhealthy. The answers are becoming clearer with more studies; however, the effectiveness of interventions to counter our self-destructive nature is more challenging.

Part 2 (chapter 3–5) provides the psychological benefits of physical activity, a critique of existing theories and models related to health behavior change, and empirical (research) support for the Disconnected Values Model.

Part 3 (chapters 6–11) consists of an explanation of each component of the DVM and takes readers through the model's application. The model should be followed in its proper sequence and in accordance with each numbered chapter.

Part 4 (chapters 12–13) addresses the understudied and challenging area of exercise (and other habits) adherence. There is content, rarely covered in the literature, on the difference between adherence and compliance. Steps to achieve and measure exercise adherence are included.

Part 5 (chapters 14–16) addresses the proper use of cognitive and behavioral strategies that promote healthy habits, particularly exercise. This content is not often addressed in the exercise psychology literature.

Part 6 (chapters 17–20) is concerned with the personal characteristics that promote and inhibit healthy habits. Certain dispositions make us more impervious to life's storms, while other dispositions produce dysfunctional behavior and can actually facilitate using unhealthy habits. Chapter 20, in particular, provides sample applications of the DVM that allow readers to view how a program is implemented.

The book concludes with two Appendices. Appendix A includes a 11-page workbook used in actual intervention sessions, taking the reader—and client—through the model one step at a time. Forms should be completed as clients go through the stages in the proper sequence. Appendix B consists of an "Exerciser Checklist," which lists the many ways exercisers should prepare for and engage in an exercise session. Exercise is a science, so there are proper procedures that should be followed to maximize exercise benefits.

The writer is indebted to Ms. Georgette Enriquez, Routledge editor, for her superb support and suggestions throughout the development and completion of this book.

Mark H. Anshel

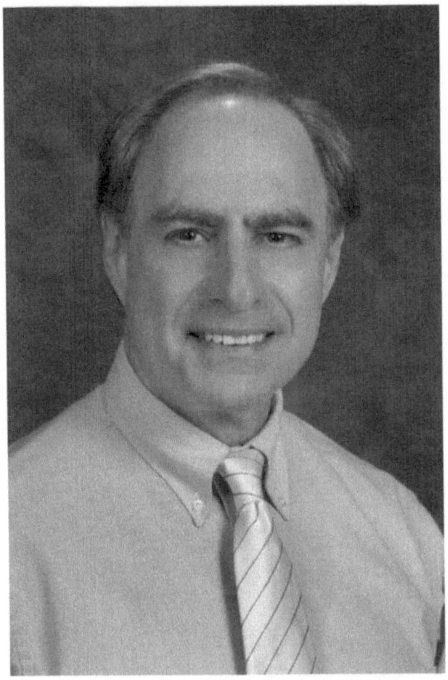

PART I

The Need to Change Health Behavior

1

EXPLAINING THE CAUSES OF UNHEALTHY HABITS

Our Self-Destructive Nature

Our unhealthy habits are catching up with us, both individually and culturally. It is more important than ever to acknowledge our self-destructive and unhealthy lifestyles and attempt to change them. The financial and personal costs of these so-called "bad habits" are extreme. We cannot make these changes alone, however. We need specialists, such as exercise and diet coaches and mental health professionals, who can show us the way, help us understand reasons for our self-destructive behavior, and help us support our new lifestyle.

Changing the thoughts, emotions, and behaviors of others is a very difficult, sometimes impossible, task. Fitness coaches, registered dieticians, even personal physicians try to influence their client's/patient's habits, often to no avail. Most of us need what is called "social support" to replace our unhealthy habits with more desirable, healthier rituals. We need to change our self-destructive behaviors and make more prudent lifestyle choices. Easier said than done, as supported by empirical research (e.g., see a review by Hall & Fong, 2007) and the extensive experience of this writer in applied settings.

Our Self-Destructive Nature

Why do we—around the world but especially in Western nations—consciously engage in behaviors that we know are unhealthy and simply bad for us? We make the decision to consume food, often in the absence of hunger; to eat in response to certain emotions rather than strictly for reasons of hunger; and to consciously refrain from engaging in regular physical activity. This is why so many of us need "experts" to tell us what to eat and how and when to exercise, to obtain the motivation to live a healthy lifestyle from our medical practitioners and (to lesser extent) from our religious leaders, and to develop routines that provide the daily structure to maintain good health. One source of our motivation to engage in healthy habits is friends and professionals, collectively referred to as *social support* (Wills & Shinar, 2000).

Most of us function better and are more likely to carry out healthy habits in the company or due to the support of others. Examples include an exercise partner, a personal trainer, a dietician, or a mental health professional; we need someone to whom we feel accountable, whose company motivates us to carry out the rituals of a healthy lifestyle, or individuals we trust to remind us to do the right thing. Coaches help others to develop and carry out various routines so that, over time, the client performs these functions independently, a process *called self-regulation*.

Based on their published model about the causes of health behavior, Professors Peter Hall and Jeffrey Fong (2007) from the University of Waterloo in Ontario, Canada, have concluded that our self-destructive nature is primarily based on two factors. First, people compare the "costs" and "benefits" of a given action, and if the benefits outweigh the costs and consequences of an action, they are more likely to take the "preferred" action. Thus, in response to hunger, boredom, or some emotion, eating a bag of French fries or ice cream minutes before bedtime satisfies hunger, tastes good, and is reasonably inexpensive—all benefits but all unhealthy. Second, the benefits of an unhealthy habit are experienced very quickly—sometimes immediately (e.g., satisfying hunger, inexpensive)—while the short-term costs (e.g., indigestion, poor sleep, weight gain) and long-term consequences (e.g., heart disease, obesity, type 2 diabetes) are much longer-term outcomes than filling up before bedtime. Because we are a culture that condones and demands immediate gratification, culturally we take the route that leads to rapid satisfaction. "Besides," many overweight people have told me, "my whole family is overweight."

As Hall and Fong (2007, p. 6) explain:

> Behaviors judged to be maladaptive in the long-run are usually driven by a strongly favorable balance of immediate costs and benefits. That is, many "maladaptive" behaviors are associated with substantial long-term costs and few (if any) long-term benefits; however, these same behaviors are frequently associated with many benefits and few costs for the individual at the time of action. In contrast, many avoided behaviors that seem "adaptive" to the outside observer (e.g., consuming raw vegetables) are, in fact, associated with substantial costs (and few benefits) at the time of actions, leading to the perplexing but common state of affairs where individuals know "what is good for them," but do not do it.

Thus, perhaps the most compelling reason why we tend to avoid health protective behaviors would be in response to these longer-term considerations (Hall & Fong, 2003). This book addresses the ways that future and current health care providers, fitness and diet coaches, and mental health professionals can combat the challenges of overcoming resistance to following proper behavior patterns and combat their addiction of immediate gratification. Most health protective behaviors, such as proper eating habits, applying sunscreen, driving within the speed limit (or slower in inclement weather), exercising regularly, and not smoking, involve inconvenience and sometimes discomfort, embarrassment, and additional expense. Some of these habits have addictive properties.

Challenges of Changing Health Behavior

As researchers have repeatedly shown, habits are very difficult to break, even unhealthy ones. Simply informing a person about the ill effects of their undesirable behavioral tendencies (e.g., late-night eating, smoking, reducing high-fat foods, the inability to cope with chronic stress, ingesting mind-altering drugs) will not necessarily result in behavior change. Study after study on the effects of educational programs on replacing unhealthy (e.g., smoking, alcohol, anabolic steroids) or illegal behaviors (e.g., manufacturing or ingesting mind-altering drugs, committing a crime) have shown that providing educational materials, lectures, and even the words of a person's medical practitioner or religious leader will not necessarily result in long-term changes in attitudes or behaviors about the negative habit. A person's self-destructive actions are better explained by the "culture" of a person's peer group, the person's self-esteem, or evidence of psychopathology (e.g., chronic depression, anxiety, emotional eating, irrational thinking). Thus, merely increasing a person's knowledge about the negative consequences of a certain habit will not necessarily result in the long-term change of that habit. What is more likely to influence behavior change and to reduce the likelihood of continued self-destructive actions? One approach is to stay positive.

Instead of associating maladaptive behaviors with poor health, Loehr and Schwartz (2003) take a more positive approach. In their intervention work with corporate clients, the author-practitioners associate healthy habits with improved energy and superior performance. These are outcomes with which most people can identify. The authors assert that unhealthy habits reduce a person's physical and mental energy. Proper eating, for instance, promotes positive emotions and heightened mental focus, which are linked to the person's sense of purpose about what he or she considers truly important (e.g., family relationships, success and effectiveness in the workplace, a strong spiritual life).

The challenge of mental and physical health care professionals, then, is to help patients/clients create four possible situations that will promote health behavior change: (1) the person experiences continued short-term benefits and/or positive feedback on certain behaviors (e.g., favorable scores on a medical or fitness test; encouraging words from a fitness coach, dietician, or medical practitioner), which will eventually lead—perhaps over a period of weeks—to a new habit of the desirable behaviors (e.g., eating an easily digestible snack while avoiding full meals if hungry before bedtime); (2) providing conditions that will facilitate the person's continuation of this favorable behavior pattern (e.g., social support, referring the person to a specialist or expert for "coaching"; (3) providing extensive and meaningful evidence of the eventual consequences of the negative, unhealthy habit (e.g., testimony of a cancer-stricken person who smoked for many years, an athlete whose health suffered from prolonged ingestion of steroids, a chronic smoker suffering from emphysema, photos and stories of drivers killed due to alcohol intake or speeding); and (4) promoting evidence of favorable outcomes from replacing the negative (unhealthy) behavior with a positive (healthy) one.

How does a mental health professional or coach successfully prevent, stop, initiate, or maintain specific behavior patterns to improve one's health and quality of life? How do we overcome the propensity of careless and toxic behaviors by individuals who do not comprehend the long-term consequences of their actions and, therefore, do not tend to take responsibility for them? What about the person who suffers from mental illness, such as clinical depression, chronic anxiety, and irrational thinking, and who "explains away" the self-destructive behavior patterns, in which the long-term consequences of these actions are irrelevant, rationalized, or not recognized? Answering these questions represents the focus of this book. Let's begin the process of obtaining these answers by defining some important concepts.

Health is a positive state of physical, mental, and social well-being, not simply the absence of injury or disease that varies over time along a continuum from wellness to illness or injury (Sarafino & Smith, 2011). *Health psychology* is a field of study and practice concerned with understanding the psychological, behavioral, and social factors that predict, describe, and determine an individual's health status, ranging from good health to illness, physically and mentally. Researchers have known for many years, for example, that smoking and other forms of tobacco use results in heart disease, compromises the immune system, and promotes different types of cancers. Clinical depression reduces energy and promotes thoughts of suicide and other forms of irrational thinking. Diet is now thought to influence attention deficit hyperactivity disorder (ADHD) and age of starting menarche among children and preadolescents.

Applied health psychology is first defined by understanding the concept of *health*, then by reviewing the concept of psychology, and finally by determining how the psychological factors that affect health have implications in real-world settings. These implications include examining how environmental and situational factors influence a person's mental and physical well-being and how practitioners (e.g., mental health professionals, medical practitioners, fitness/nutrition/life coaches) can influence the individual's health, well-being, and quality of life. At the core of applied health psychology is the attempt to understand, prevent, manage, and, if possible, eradicate the onset of mental and physical disease (Anshel, 2014).

Health psychologists attempt to promote a person's mental and physical health by: (1) understanding the personal and situational factors that explain a person's health or illness; (2) favorably influencing the individual's mental state by understanding the causes of dysfunctional or maladaptive behavioral patterns (i.e., "bad" habits that negatively influence health and well-being); (3) preventing or treating illness through the use of various forms of therapy and interventions; (4) identifying the psychological, behavioral, and situational factors that explain a person's illness or dysfunction; and (5) determining the effects of cognitive and behavioral strategies on improving mental and physical health and quality of life.

Use of the title (and credential) "health psychologist" infers that the individual is a licensed clinical or counseling psychologist with a specialization in understanding the personal (i.e., a person's thoughts, emotions, personality traits) and environmental factors (i.e., psycho-social stress, relationships) that may explain a person's physical and mental condition. In addition, health psychologists are interactive with medical practitioners, rehabilitation and physical therapists, dieticians, personal trainers/exercise coaches, and other specialists whose expertise will accompany the array of services and expertise needed to provide proper counsel and intervention strategies.

While the content of this book addresses changes in health behavior, among the most common and important behavior patterns is exercise. Readers will notice this emphasis but should be able to transfer this material to other unhealthy behaviors, such as poor diet and improper eating habits, smoking, tobacco use, in general, poor sleep, excessive stress, poor coping skills, and others. Table 1.1 outlines the various definitions related to health and exercise.

"Wellness," a more global concept, is usually defined as a generalized state of good health, the optimal soundness of body and mind. More specifically, wellness is "the achievement of the highest level of health possible in physical, social, intellectual, emotional, environmental, and spiritual dimensions" (Hopson, Donatelle, & Littrell, 2009, p. 2). "Wellness" and "health" are often used interchangeably. Wellness has several dimensions, and the dimension that is most closely allied with this book is physical wellness. To Hopson et al., physical wellness consists of "all aspects of a sound body, including body size and shape, sensory sharpness and responsiveness, body functioning, physical strength, flexibility and endurance, resistance to diseases and disorders, and recuperative abilities" (p. 4). One subdimension of physical wellness is physical fitness.

Physical fitness is the ability of the human organism to function efficiently and effectively (Corbin & Lindsey, 1994). Because physical fitness is a very important outcome of engaging in exercise and other forms of physical activity, mental health professionals, as well as others who counsel in the health field, should help clients/patients achieve better fitness through an array of strategies that will be discussed in this book. The benefits of engaging in regular physical activity, particularly exercise, is enormous, and getting clients/patients to increase their level of physical activity should be a primary outcome of the counseling process.

Researchers have designated five subdimensions, or measures, of physical fitness. These are *cardiorespiratory endurance* (also called "aerobic fitness"), which

TABLE 1.1 Definitions of dimensions and subdimensions of health and wellness

Health: a positive state of physical, mental, and social well-being	**Wellness:** a generalized state of good health and the optimal soundness of body and mind
Health Psychology: a field of study and practice concerned with understanding the psychological, behavioral, and social factors that predict, describe, and determine an individual's health status	**Physical Wellness:** all aspects of a sound body, including body size and shape, sensory sharpness and responsiveness, body functioning, physical strength, flexibility and endurance, resistance to diseases and disorders, and recuperative abilities
Applied Health Psychology: a field of study and practice concerned with examining how environmental and situational factors influence a person's mental and physical well-being and how practitioners (e.g., mental health professionals/health psychologists, fitness and nutrition coaches) influence the individual's health, well-being, and quality of life	**Physical Fitness:** ability of the human organism to function efficiently and effectively. Includes cardiorespiratory endurance (aerobic fitness), muscular strength, muscular endurance, flexibility, and body composition
Health Psychologist: a licensed clinical psychologist with a specialization in understanding the personal and environmental factors that may explain a person's physical and mental condition	**Exercise Psychology*:** the study of psychological factors underlying participation in and adherence to physical activity programs

*There is no formal or legal recognition, at this time, of the professional titles "exercise psychologist" or "fitness psychologist." However, a licensed psychologist who is credentialed in the state (or Canadian province) in which he or she practices may use either of these terms to describe an area of specialization or expertise.

focuses on improved function of the heart and lungs; *muscular strength*; *muscular endurance*; *flexibility*; and *body composition* (also referred to as "percent body fat"). Hopson et al. (2009) further define *health-related components of physical fitness* as "components of physical fitness that have a relationship with good health" (p. 31).

One form of achieving better physical fitness is a type of physical activity called "exercise." Different forms of exercise achieve each of the five types of physical fitness. Why some individuals choose to exercise, while others do not, and how practitioners can improve exercise participation and maintenance are just a small segment of a field that deals with the relationship between the mental and emotional factors that explain exercise behavior; this relationship is called "exercise psychology."

Exercise psychology is defined in *The Dictionary of the Sport and Exercise Sciences* (Anshel et al., 1991) as "the study of psychological factors underlying participation and adherence in physical activity programs" (p. 56). Researchers have determined that, for instance, exercise alters mood, reduces stress, reduces the effects of mental disorders such as depression and anxiety, and improves self-confidence and self-esteem. Other studies have shown that regular cardiovascular exercise increases energy, improves tolerance to acute and chronic pain, and enhances quality of life. Helping clients increase their intensity and frequency of exercise is an important outcome of health counseling.

Researchers in applied health and exercise psychology also want to know the personal and situational factors that explain, even predict, the reasons some individuals begin and adhere to an exercise habit (or any other form of regular physical activity such as biking, hiking, skiing, and sport participation), while others do not develop this habit and, in fact, have an aversion to physical activity. Is one's attitude toward exercise related to childhood or adolescent experiences in former physical education classes or coaches who burned out their former athletes with excessive physical training and conditioning? Along these lines, why do some individuals adhere to their exercise program while others quit—often within the first three to six months after starting a new program rather than adopting a lifelong habit? What psychological issues might impede a person's decision to begin and maintain an exercise program? It is well known that conditions collectively called *psychopathology*, or mental illness, strongly influence a person's energy and willingness to exercise regularly. Examples include chronic (long-term) forms of stress, depression, and anxiety; irrational thinking (e.g., "I don't deserve to be fit/thinner/more attractive/healthy"); emotional eating; low self-esteem; low confidence; fear of failure; and high somatic, or physical, anxiety (i.e., a person's worry about his or her physical appearance).

Changing a person's well-learned habits is among the most challenging objective in the health care industry. As the results of studies tell us more and more about the very expensive and undesirable long-term effects of an unhealthy lifestyle, and the importance and benefits of "healthy living" becomes increasingly clear, an emerging need to provide professional services to meet needs of the general public has evolved. This process is best met by generating new approaches to instructing future professionals in novel and creative ways to change health behavior. This process is best reflected in the field of applied health psychology.

The *Healthy People 2010* report, published by the U.S. Department of Health and Human Services (USDHHS; 2000), indicated that only 22% of adults in the United States engage in physical activity of relatively moderate to light intensity for 30 minutes five or more times a week. Almost 25% of the population is completely sedentary. For those who begin a regular exercise program, up to 50% will drop out within the first six months. We are eating more, exercising less, and getting fatter; about two-thirds of the U.S. population is overweight or obese. Thus, there is what's commonly called an obesity epidemic, and the current state of the nation's health is costing 17% of the nation's overall budget, or several billion dollars. An overweight employee costs employers $5,000 more a year in health costs than a healthy-weight individual, according to a survey by the National Business Group on Health (*USA Today*, 11/25/11, p. 2A).

There is plenty of blame to go around for this sad state of affairs. Our school physical education classes either no longer exist, consist of "free play" rather than fitness coaching, or focus on learning and performing sports skills, again avoiding exercise as a primary component of the course. To make matters worse, students in PE classes are often criticized for their less-than-stellar performance during sports competition; teachers use exercise as a form of punishment; and sports coaches tend to overtrain their athletes, resulting in exercise burnout and a negative attitude toward exercise. The result is that athletes stop becoming physically active when they retire from sports. Other reasons for weight gain as we age include being obsessed with food and feeling a disdain for exercise and other forms of physical activity. The consequence of these attitudes and behavioral patterns is an increase rate of type 2 diabetes, usually attributed to obesity, and various diseases.

The role of applied health psychology, of which exercise psychology is one component, is particularly important in forming a conceptual framework and creating a structure and a field of research and practice that promotes a healthy lifestyle. Exercise psychology complements the areas of health psychology and exercise science area that are collectively devoted to understanding the physiological and psychological effects of exercise on the person. Exercise psychology addresses the effects of interventions that influence exercise participation and adherence.

The focus of this book, then, is to provide guidelines for applying the Disconnected Values Model to assist mental health professionals and others whose focus is to change the health behavior of their clients or patients. This includes individuals in the health care industry, including medical practitioners, fitness coaches, mental health professionals, registered dieticians, sports coaches, physical education teachers, rehabilitation specialists executive/lifestyle coaches, and anyone concerned with helping people learn and apply new routines that will improve their health, energy, and quality of life. Another important, perhaps primary, focus of this book is to improve fitness and quality of life among clients. Chapter 2 addresses the perplexing question about why we do things every single day that we know are bad for us and how to replace our self-destructive actions with life-enhancing and health-promoting routines.

There are many ethical issues that accompany a new and growing area of study and practice. Issues that need to be resolved include discovering who "owns" the emerging field of health behavior change. What credentials are needed to practice in this area, and what professional organizations best represent this area of study and practice? Like all areas of academic and practice, proper ethics is imperative. The use of titles, requisite skills needed to practice and obtain funds from clients, and the ability to be current in the scientific literature and to apply that knowledge all need to be monitored by a professional credentialing body, not unlike most areas of practice (e.g., medicine, mental health, education).

There is an emerging field called "health fitness psychology" that has many masters. Who is the so-called rightful owner of this field? Multiple fields of study and practice have contributed to fitness psychology, including various components of psychology (e.g., clinical, counseling, cognitive, health), exercise and sport science, and sports medicine. At some point, one of these disciplines, all recognized internationally as reputable, scholarly, and with an applied component, will need to step forward and more clearly define and coordinate the boundaries, educational background, skills, qualifications, credentials, and types of programs that represent the field.

Changing one's own routines, however unhealthy and self-destructive, is extraordinarily difficult because routines represent our comfort zone; we say, "I've always done it that way." Or we justify our unhealthy habits by refusing to perceive that a problem to our health exists. I have often heard obese individuals assert that "my medical test scores are fine so I do not have a problem." We are in a constant state of denial that is partially based on the absence of dangerous signs of poor health from test scores, a personal care provider failing to point out health concerns, claims that "good health runs in my family" (e.g., "My grandmother smoked for years and lived to the age of 85"), and—my favorite—"Well, you gotta die of something."

Having an "outsider" (e.g., fitness coach, registered dietician, health care worker, mental health professional) attempt to replace well-entrenched unhealthy habits with healthier, more desirable routines is even more difficult and challenging. This book introduces a novel, client-centered approach to helping others replace their unhealthy habits with more desirable routines by integrating the concept of values into their daily thinking and asking them to rethink the benefits, costs, and consequences of their current lifestyle.

References

Anshel, M. H. (2014). *Applied health fitness psychology*. Champaign, IL: Human Kinetics.

Anshel, M. H., Freedson, P., Hamill, J., Haywood, K., Horvat, M., & Plowman, S. A. (1991). *Dictionary of the sport and exercise sciences*. Champaign, IL: Human Kinetics.

Corbin, C. B., & Lindsey, R. (1994). *Concepts of physical fitness with laboratories* (8th ed.). Dubuque, IA: Wm. C. Brown Communications.

Hall, P. A., & Fong, G. T. (2003). The effects of a brief time perspective intervention for increasing physical activity among young adults. *Psychology and Health, 18*, 685–706.

Hall, P. A., & Fong, G. T. (2007). Temporal self-regulation theory: A model for individual health behavior. *Health Psychology Review, 1*, 6–52.

Hopson, J. L., Donatelle, R. J., & Littrell, T. R. (2009). *Get fit, stay well.* San Francisco: Benjamin-Cummings.

Loehr, J., & Schwartz, T. (2003). *The power of full engagement: Managing energy, not time, is the key to high performance and personal renewal.* New York: Free Press.

Sarafino, E. P., & Smith, T. W. (2011). *Health psychology: Biopsychosocial interactions* (7th ed.). Hoboken, NJ: Wiley.

Wills, T. A., & Shinar, O. (2000). Measuring perceived and received social support. In S. Cohen, L. G. Underwood, & B. H. Gottlieb (Eds.), *Social support measurement and intervention* (pp. 86–135). New York: Oxford University Press.

2

CHALLENGES OF CHANGING HEALTH BEHAVIOR

Changing habits is among the most complex and difficult tasks we can attempt. One reason for this is because habits have become automatic and comfortable over time. They are entrenched in our daily rituals and perceived as beneficial to our life. If the negative consequences of our habits were more pronounced and apparent then the benefits, it is more likely we would rethink performing many of these habits. It is especially challenging when the source of motivation to change is external (i.e., a coach, mental health professional, parent, friend, teacher, or mentor), rather than when the need to change is generated within. When the source for changing behavior is external, it is referred to as *extrinsic motivation*. When the source is self-induced and initiated, it is called *intrinsic motivation*. These sources of motivation will be discussed at length later in the chapter. Helping others change their self-destructive—but comfortable—behavior patterns that are directly linked to one's health and well-being is the focus of this book.

It's imperative that mental health professionals, health educators, personal trainers (coaches), registered dieticians, medical practitioners (e.g., physicians, nurses), life/executive coaches, and anyone else concerned with health behavior change be able to use the proper strategies for increasing a person's sense of urgency in changing some feature of his or her current lifestyle. Perhaps one of the bigger challenges facing these professionals is helping clients or patients feel the need for changing their well-established habits.

Unless individuals feel that beginning a new habit or stopping an old one is in their best interest, changing unhealthy habits will not occur. People need to feel that their current level of some undesirable personal characteristic they want to improve upon (e.g., fitness, body weight, medical condition, appearance, mental condition—depression, anxiety) warrants a lifestyle change that will improve on that situation. The incentive to change a habit can be externally imposed but for a relatively short period of time. It is far more desirable to enable the person to *want* or feel the *need* to change. A change in a health-related ritual, or negative habit, is an active, not passive, process that requires self-motivation and energy. The primary source of energy is derived internally and is the genesis of a process called *motivation*.

Motivation and Changing Health Behavior

Motivating a person to perform an activity she or she already enjoys—let's say convincing a person to attend a restaurant with a very good reputation—may seem to be a relatively easy task. It is far more challenging, however, to provide a person with the incentive to do something that is contrary to their usual routine or habit. This is particularly the case if the client and the professional have not established a relationship based on trust and mutual respect. Researchers and practitioners have attempted to identify the factors that provide the ignition—the spark—that will promote health behavior change. This has been particularly challenging when the behavior change runs counter to the individual's past experiences and does not carry immediate or short-term benefits. Examples include feeling the benefits of a new exercise program, detecting and feeling better due to a change in eating habits, and improving sleep patterns that results in improved mood and work productivity. Changing a person's routines and habits are very difficult and often accompanied by dropping out and lack of long-term adherence.

The question must be asked concerning doing the things we know will help us feel better, provide more energy, and improve our long-term physical and mental health and physical appearance: Why is motivation even necessary? Why are some individuals self-motivated to "do the right thing," and have the knowledge and incentive to look after their health? In order to develop effective interventions to promote new, healthier habits, it is important to discuss the antecedents of low motivation to develop rituals and behavior patterns that are "healthy" and bring us enormous benefits. Perhaps there is no better example of a poor habit than our tendency to avoid regular exercise and other forms of physical activity. There are some reasons that might explain our sedentary lifestyle, even when we "know" that exercise is a very important part of maintaining good health. Understanding the sources of our disdain for exercise, at least in selected countries, begins our journey to provide interventions that change these negative attitudes and self-destructive behavior patterns into healthier, more desirable habits. To obtain theoretical and applied information about intrinsic and extrinsic motivation, readers are referred to the book edited by Martin Haggar and Nikos Chatzisarantis (2007) located in the reference list.

Reasons for Negative Attitudes toward Exercise

What has happened to us over the years as we grew older? As children, we would spend hours after school engaged in some sort of physical activity; we called it "play." Children and adolescents today are far less active than past generations. Yes, there are more options for school-aged youth today that require sitting rather than moving, but explanations for a sedentary lifestyle are more complex than sitting at computers, toying with cell phones and iPads, and staying home when mom and dad are out working. Somewhere along the way, we forgot the joys and needs to be physically active. Our reduced wish for physical activity and sedentary alternatives turned "play" into "work."

Compared to past decades, adults have also stopped enjoying physical activity. Positive attitudes toward exercise, sports participation, and other forms of physical activity have become increasingly negative. Our preferred sedentary lifestyle, combined with consuming massive amounts of food, has resulted in excessive weight gain and, sadly, weight-related diseases such as Type 2 diabetes and various types of cancer. Below are several likely reasons for the turnaround in attitude—from positive to negative—toward exercise, with direct implications for other unhealthy habits and acting in ways that run counter to our best interests and health. Therapists and health coaches should be able to apply these factors to other unhealthy habits.

Experience in school physical education (PE). While more research is needed in this area, it is apparent that many of our students have had negative experiences in their school physical education classes—elementary, middle, and secondary school levels. Reasons abound. For instance, as O'Rourke (2011) found, better-skilled individuals are picked to participate on sports teams as part of PE class, while less-skilled individuals are left out. In addition, learning sport skills is often replaced by "free play," in which students are asked to participate in various sports on their own. Individuals with limited sport skills, less motor coordination, or who are overweight, however, are ignored, criticized, or teased. Further, many PE programs have no—or limited—fitness components, including an absence of fitness testing and exercise training, that would allow the students to improve their fitness scores and to get in better physical condition. No wonder the desire to develop a positive attitude toward physical activity and exercise is lacking. The lack of exercise is leading to terribly high rates of childhood and adolescent obesity and Type 2 diabetes and resulting in poor health, astronomical health care costs, and a shortened lifespan.

Exercise burnout. Burnout is characterized by feelings of emotional exhaustion and a reduced sense of personal accomplishment about one's work (Maslach & Jackson, 1981). These characteristics may be applied to exercise, in which a person feels physically and emotionally drained of energy and motivation. Being required to exercise, especially at high intensity levels that risk experiencing injury or illness, common among highly skilled athletes, may result in exercise burnout. In sport, this outcome is referred to as *overtraining*.

Exercise as punishment. The so-called "tradition" of using exercise as a form of punishment (e.g., "You were absent from practice; that will cost you 20 push-ups"; "We lost so take 10 laps around the field") results in a deep disdain for exercise. When exercise is used as a form of punishment, we are associating exercise with punishment and unpleasant feelings. We then spend our life perceiving exercise and other forms of physical activity as sometime to be avoided. Physical activity should not be associated with undesirable behavior.

Lack of fitness knowledge. Gaining the benefits of participating in a program of regular exercise or other forms of physical activity requires knowing the correct technique; exercise is a science that requires proper techniques that must be. These techniques must be learned through proper instruction by a specialist, often requiring payment to a personal trainer or coach. Failure to use the proper techniques may result in injury and the lack of fitness improvement.

Unpleasant feelings; higher perceived effort. Because most of us lead sedentary lives, our body is not "trained" for more vigorous levels of physical activity; we struggle with bouts of high exercise intensity, making physical exertion unpleasant. These feelings are exacerbated if the person is overweight or obese. Our physiology—heart rate, respiration rate, hormonal activity—will eventually adapt to the stress of vigorous physical activity and exertion. Only by placing physical demands on our body can we experience what is called a "training effect."

Common Barriers to Exercise Participation

There are reasons, good and bad, valid and invalid, that explain a person's decision to engage or not engage in an unhealthy habit. Similar to the previous list, lack of regular exercise will serve as the template for barriers to most of our unhealthy habits. Here are the most common and, for some people, "valid" exercise barriers.

Not enough time. Starting a new habit—exercise, changes in eating patterns, or improving sleep quality, among many others—requires time and patience. With sufficient time and motivation, changes in behavior patterns—new habits—become automatic. Taking exercise as an example, one of the most common reasons people give for not exercising regularly is lack of time (Hellston & Rogers, 2009). But is lack of time *really* a valid excuse?

Let's do the math. There are 168 hours in a week (7 days x 24 hours/day). The exercise physiology literature indicates that cardiovascular and strength fitness should occur about three hours per week. Three hours is just 1.5% of the full week (168 hours). Therefore, it takes *less* time to improve fitness than most of us use our cell phones, iPads, or watch television. It may be argued, then, that lack of time is a mere *perception* for providing an excuse not to exercise. Exercise, like any other habit, can become an integral part of one's daily routine, rather than a behavior a person performs "when I have the time." Time management skills are needed to "fit in" a new ritual.

Convenience/availability. Workout facilities or programs that are perceived as "conveniently located" are more likely to attract exercisers than facilities or programs that are perceived as out of the way, inconvenient, or not compatible with the exerciser's goals. Facilities and programs that are available and of relatively close proximity to the exerciser that will foster participation in and adherence to the new habit, in this example, exercise (Sallis & Owen, 1999).

Injury. Injury may become one outcome of engaging in regular exercise, but it is also self-destructive to exercise if already injured. Tissue damage can become more extensive and the level of discomfort can be excessive. In addition, unfit individuals have a lower pain threshold than their more fit counterparts. The bottom line here is to "listen to your body"; if there is pain or extreme discomfort—not just muscle stiffness, which is a common outcome of vigorous physical activity among unfit individuals—rest until the discomfort goes away.

Boredom or lack of enjoyment. For many individuals, particularly the unfit, physical activity is both unpleasant and unexciting. This is one reason to explain exercise dropout and is an impediment to developing any healthy habit. An unfit, often overweight individual who exercises alone (e.g., walking, riding a stationary bicycle, lifting weights) may feel very much alone and uninspired; exercise becomes an unpleasant experience. Because so few exercise beginners recruit a performance coach, are given proper instruction, or exercise with encouraging friends, it is no wonder the dropout rate for exercise novices is so high.

Excessive or unachievable goals. It is not uncommon to set goals related to developing a new habit. The problem is that goal setting is a science, and too many individuals set goals that are excessive and unrealistic. Exercise novices, for instance, want to engage in new exercise or dietary habits that will result in physical features that are more fantasy than reality. In fact, a goal such as losing an extensive amount of weight in a relatively short time due to a new exercise program or diet regimen may be—and have been—potentially fatal. Setting goals related to starting a new healthy habit should include the insights of a professional such as an exercise coach, registered dietician, medical provider, or mental health professional.

Research in the exercise physiology literature indicates that four to six weeks is needed to markedly improve fitness after beginning an exercise program (Corbin & Lindsey, 1994). This also marks the time frame when significantly improved fitness will increase, while exercise exertion and physical fatigue will feel less intense. Therefore, health professionals want to encourage their clients to exercise at least three times a week for four weeks so that they can begin to notice more pleasant, fewer undesirable side effects from physical exertion. Other habits also require a minimal time frame before the habit becomes automatic, resulting in a lifestyle change.

Lack of instruction and coaching. New habits almost always require new knowledge and the input of experts. Sleep clinics and their staff are able to diagnose sleep disorders, some of which can be fatal, such as severe sleep apnea (i.e., temporary cessation of breathing). Mental health professionals and registered dieticians can detect eating disorders, and physiotherapists can help patients overcome joint pain through therapeutic exercise. Obtaining a new habit should almost always involve an expert who can provide proper testing, instruction, and coaching that, taken together, will more likely result in treatment adherence and a successful addition of the new habit to one's lifestyle.

Perceived lack of improvement. Having a sense of achievement and improvement is intrinsic to our personality, especially in Western cultures. A person's willingness to replace an unhealthy habit with a healthy one, and then to persist in that changed (improved) habit, is often based on the perception of improved changes in some important aspect of life. Examples include weight (fat) loss, exercising at reduced exertion and discomfort, superior performance outcomes, and improved test scores. This is why exercise pretesting, to establish a fitness baseline prior to starting a program, has long-term motivational value.

Absence of social support. Social support is a very powerful type of influence of human behavior. Lox et al. (2014) define social support as "the perceived comfort, caring, assistance, and information that a person receives from others" (p. 101). Examples of social support include verbal and nonverbal positive reinforcement from partners, family, and friends (e.g., "Well done, Sue"); exercising with a friend; being encouraged by others to maintain a certain habit or behavior; obtaining instruction or coaching; or exercising under generally pleasant and comfortable conditions. Considerable research has shown that social support in exercise settings has high motivational value and results in better short-term and long-term adherence to an exercise habit, as opposed to little or no social support.

Taken together, there is no shortage of barriers that will prevent individuals from starting or maintaining a change in one or more health behaviors, for example, engaging in a regular exercise program. Each of the issues listed earlier can apply to other health behaviors, both physical (e.g., sleep quality, dietary and nutritional habits, tobacco and alcohol use, improved communication) and emotional/mental (e.g., impatience, anger, effective vs. ineffective coping with stress, improved concentration, maintaining emotional control).

Mental health professionals are in a position to help their clients acknowledge their undesirable, unhealthy habits and to replace them with lifestyle choices that will bring enormous happiness, energy, satisfaction, and improved health, both mental and physical. The mental health professional can fit the role of a client's performance coach by providing the person with insights into their behaviors, the "benefits," short-term costs, and long-term consequences of their selected habits, and provide information and strategies to overcome resistance to behavior change, especially behaviors related to one's health. Sometimes ongoing community programs can be recommended such as a weight-reducing program, a local fitness club/center, groups that cater to specific behavioral problems (e.g., alcohol or drug abuse programs/clinics), and referrals to local specialists and experts. Often, people are driven to changing behaviors based on undesirable test scores; people are often driven by numbers. Testing, or "pre testing and post-testing," is one source of motivation toward behavior change.

Applying Motivation Theory in Health Behavior Change

What is clear across all types, categories, and theories of motivation, however, is that behavior cannot be intentional, learning cannot occur, information cannot be processed, and changing health behavior cannot be initiated and maintained without motivation. The "direction" of motivation refers to the target in which the individual is moving, and where one's energy is being directed. The motivated exerciser is energized to engage in a task that the person finds meaningful, in our example, engaging in physical activity or some other healthy habit. Motivation, therefore, is a conscious, active, and purposeful process. Motivated behavior requires conscious thought and planning.

Sometimes motivated behavior is a reaction to aversive (undesirable) consequences. Forcing someone to exerciser—let's say as a form of punishment in sport settings or to "push" an exerciser in a fitness class—has the very undesirable effect of instilling negative attitudes toward exercise, fitness, and physical training. These threats usually lead to motivated behaviors because they are controlled by their connections to consequences. However, because these actions represent a negative approach to motivation, they have a relatively short-term effect, as opposed to the preferred long-term, even permanent behavior change. Even better would be long-term consequences of exercise-improved fitness, more energy, better health, and superior performance.

A far superior value of motivation for changing health behavior is to encourage the person (client) to maintain positive feelings about the new habit that accompanies the new behavior. Acknowledging the benefits of a new habit improve the probability of long-term adherence to that habit. The secret to a long-term commitment to the new habit is called *intrinsic motivation*.

One of the most challenging motivational strategies for mental health practitioners and others who attempt to change client/patient health behavior is to determine what it takes to motivate each individual to acquire new habit(s). The process of *self-regulation* is particularly useful in helping others to conclude that increased effort will lead to meeting desirable goals (Vansteenkiste, Soenens, & Lens, 2007). The exerciser who gives 100% every week, for instance, but still physically struggles, is not detecting weight loss or improved appearance, or whose goals far exceed their capabilities will not likely be motivated to persist at the activity. These exercisers will be less motivated to give 100%, leading to feelings of helplessness about changing their fitness level or reaching some other desirable goal. The typical result is dropping out of the exercise program or stopping the new habit.

Using exercise as an example of acquiring a desirable habit, Howley and Franks (2007) suggest ways that fitness coaches can increase motivation to improve exercise adherence. One way to foster the exerciser's incentive is to point out specific ways in which following specific behaviors will lead to desirable outcomes (e.g., "If you work hard at least three times a week, you'll make faster progress than if you exercise on an irregular schedule and do not give 100%"). Exercisers can also improve their incentive to get fitter by engaging in types of exercises they find pleasant and plan to maintain week after week. Losing too much weight and having unattainable goals, on the other hand, is not realistic or desirable for most individuals. Improved fitness and weight loss, however, is far more realistic and achievable. The most important form of motivation is based on the individual's desire to perform an activity based on personal satisfaction, pleasure, even fun—*intrinsic motivation*.

Sources of Motivation

A person's motivation to act in a certain, often preplanned, and predictable manner reflects the combination of personal and situational factors. The intention of motivated behavior is to create and maintain a sense of direction, energy, drive, and incentive to meet one or more desirable goals. Sources of motivation are usually referred to as person-centered and situation-centered.

Person-Centered Motivational Sources

One way of understanding sources of motivation to maintain healthy lifestyle choices is to measure personal dispositions. It is thought that motivation sources and intensity reflect the individuals' personality traits (e.g., need achievement, self-esteem, physique anxiety, among many others), orientations/styles (e.g., need for goals, competitiveness, coping style, mental toughness), and needs (e.g., needs for recognition, approval, achievement, competence). Because motivated behavior is usually voluntary, the actions of a motivated person is often predictable. For instance, when a dental patient is informed that failure to floss at least once per day, preferably before bedtime, may result in tooth decay and eventual loss of teeth, the patient is more likely to change behavior—to floss—as opposed to not taking the habit of flossing seriously. Thus, the person-centered view of motivation is that individuals are driven to change behavior if they have the incentive to reach a goal, achieve at a high level, or experience optimal performance. Motivation cannot be forced. Individual desire is the first and foremost characteristic of motivation.

Situation-Centered Motivational Sources

A supportive environment enhances a person's motivation to perform a task or meet a goal, according to situation-centered motivation. Not surprisingly, a person's surroundings and interactions with others constantly influence the intensity of a person's motivation level. For example, exercisers are more likely to provide optimal effort if the environment in which they exercise induces feelings of safety, security, familiarity, comfort, and sufficient arousal level. Exercising in the privacy of one's home or publically, such as in a fitness club, presents conditions that may either heighten or reduce motivation level. In another example, some individuals are more motivated to exercise during certain times of the year (e.g., in warmer weather) or when transportation is available and safe (e.g., being driven to the exercise venue). Thus, the location of exercise, the type of exercises experienced, and the environment in which exercise takes place all influence an individual's exercise motivation.

There are two primary limitations of the situation-centered view of motivation. First, some situations do not influence an individual's motivation, up or down, and second, many personal factors (e.g., the individual's personal characteristics and needs) may strongly influence behavior. For instance, some situations are quite unpleasant and demotivating, yet a person may conclude that "failure is not an option" and remain motivated to achieve a particular goal. In one study, Martin Ginis, Burke, and Gauvin (2007) found that exercise novices are often *demotivated* when asked to exercise in front of mirrors, whereas more fit individuals often find mirrors motivating.

Interactive Personal and Situational Sources

The *interaction model* is a combination of personal and situational motivation sources, describing a third explanation for motivation. This model posits that motivational feelings and actions result from a combination of personal and situational factors. For example, the motivational factors that influence a person's decision to exercise combines personal factors (e.g., high self-esteem, confidence, goal orientation), situational factors (e.g., social support, such as exercising in the company of others or being encouraged), close proximity of an exercise facility to one's work or home, and desirable exercise facilities and equipment. Determining the sources of motivation to exercise is important in making exercise a lifestyle habit.

How effective is feeling threatened or other negative feelings on motivation? PE teachers, sports coaches, and medical practitioners, who divulge test results to their patients, are individuals who attempt to increase motivation through unpleasant information or, at times, intimidation. Using exercise as a form of punishment is well known among school PE teachers and sports coaches, while medical practitioners may expresses concern about the person's health status to motivate a change in behavior (e.g., dieting, starting an exercise program) to overcome poor health. Short-term threats about health status have motivational effects. It is also true that sometimes this type of treatment from an authority figure (e.g., physician, personal trainer) is desirable, even needed, to increase the exerciser's incentive to change from a sedentary to a more active lifestyle.

Reliance on negative motivational techniques, however, has two shortcomings. First, these techniques usually have only short-term effects because the exerciser's behavior changes only until the source of threat is removed (e.g., losing weight, feeling better, improving performance). As indicated earlier, after the threat is removed, the incentive to persist in this activity is minimal. This is one reason so many athletes, elite and nonelite, tend to avoid exercising after their days as sports competitors have ended.

The second shortcoming, as indicated earlier, is that threatening another person creates extrinsic, not intrinsic, incentive to change behavior. Some intrinsic value will be derived if the individual views exercise and fitness as beneficial to his or her health and quality of life and if the exercise experience is pleasant and reaffirms the person's sense of competence. Exercise can be an extrinsic motivator, however, if the sole aim is to improve fitness or physical appearance, such as an athlete who trains for competition, or to achieve some other outcome.

In summary, a person's motivation to change health behavior (e.g., increasing physical activity, changes in diet, sleep patterns, strategies to reduce stress) is dependent on meeting the individual's personal needs and objectives. At the same time, the individual wants to pursue a certain predetermined course of action and possess the necessary feelings and attitudes associated with performance success.

Antecedents and Mechanisms for Changing Health Behavior

Changing habits—even those that are very unhealthy—is very challenging for both patients/clients and practitioners. Most cardiologists, when asked how they motivate a patient to change an unhealthy habit, usually related to changes in eating and exercise habits, indicate "after the first heart attack." It often takes a tragedy, near-death experience, or threatening test result to convince people that their life is *now* at risk—not next year or in 10 years but now. Even then, some individuals are addicted to certain self-destructive habits, such as tobacco use, and will not change behavior. Emotional eating, food addictions, certain work habits that promote stress (e.g., work addiction), and other unhealthy habits may persist, even after being warned of upcoming dangers. One more source of resisting health behavior change is a person who firmly believes that his or her life is under the control of a higher power; "it's in the Lord's hands." What are the factors that may foster a person's decision to "buy in" to the need to lead a healthier life?

Develop a Treatment Strategy

Program Planning

The DVM intervention must be planned and time allocated that allows for at least most of the stages to be experienced. A second, follow-up session to discuss—at length—the action plan is usually needed. Sometimes a discussion about treatment strategy for applying the DVM can last an hour, sometimes two or even three hours. It may be carried out privately or in a group setting. Under what conditions will the intervention be carried out? Individually between therapist and client? In a group setting? If the latter, will participants also be coworkers and hear their colleagues convey very personal information?

Privacy Issues

It is imperative that DVM program leaders respect the privacy of their client/participants/patients. While it may be acceptable to ask group members from the same company or organization to experience the DVM together, it may not be acceptable that these individuals share responses to program content. It is especially important to separate management staff from their subordinates in the same program. Again, caution is required.

Program Facilities and Scheduling

Another treatment strategy concerns having the program, facilities, equipment, and support staff all scheduled in advance. Be sure that a facility is available for the program that is of sufficient size, has privacy, is available for the scheduled time of day and day of the week, is comfortable (especially seats), is equipped with proper audio-visual equipment (if needed), has pencils and paper available, includes a snack bar (if the session goes past one hour; more on this later) and water, and (if possible) has close proximity to an exercise facility where the program participants can receive exercise instruction in addition to listening to a lecture and engaging in the workshop.

Support Staff

A fourth issue concerns the availability and participation of support staff. The program may include interacting with a coach or therapist or some other professional but may also include specialists in fitness, nutrition, stress management, medical practitioners, massage therapists, or leaders with other skills, such as a nurse (perhaps to take a blood sample). Here's an example of poor program planning. A wellness-type center in Florida provides a program for corporate clients held over several days. Often, a company will send their management staff to the center to experience the full program. Group size can be anywhere from two to 30 men and women. While the lecture and workbook segment of the program can easily be given in a group setting with only one leader, the exercise segment of the program requires several staff to handle groups, in this case, a group of 15 participants. Instead, the program allowed for only two fitness coaches for this group of 15, leaving many individuals to stand around and wait for one of the coaches to instruct them on proper weight-training technique. Clients who paid a considerable sum for the three-day program were walking around and waiting. Not the best use of time or expertise due to a lack of proper staffing.

Long-Term Adherence

Many programs/seminars/lectures that promise behavior change fail to incorporate the interaction of staff with the clients/customers/patients for follow-up purposes and determine adherence to their new habits. After the program has been completed, clients will be asked to initiate at least one new habit, perhaps more than one. How long does it take to establish a new habit or routine? Studies and experts differ on this issue, but a safe range of time would be eight to 15 weeks of replacing a former unhealthy behavior with a new, more desirable ritual for the latter to become automatic. A program is more effective if the leader or appointed staff member monitors client adherence to the new ritual, offers the client remediation and emotional/spiritual support, and is available for further instruction and coaching if the client "stumbles" in adhering to the new behavior pattern. While monitoring adherence takes time, it is also needed; changing habits is often very challenging and sometimes impossible without additional coaching. Part 4 (chapters 12–14) of this book further discusses approaches to improving client long-term adherence to new health rituals.

In summary, the DVM is an intervention that requires sufficient time, privacy, confidentiality, planning, and interactions between the leader/professional and client, either in private/individual or group settings, and a plan to maintain client contact after the program to insure or at least to promote long-term adherence to the new ritual(s).

Determine the Behavior for Change

Perhaps the initial stage of health behavior change is to acknowledge the specific behavior the client wishes to change. Rollnick, Mason, and Butler (1999) suggest the most common behaviors that practitioners need to address (paraphrased and edited):

- Eating (less, different items, adjust timing of meals);
- Drinking (less alcohol, abstaining altogether, fewer soft drinks);
- Physical activity (more exercise, specific types of activity);
- Smoking (fewer cigarettes, abstain altogether, refrain from all tobacco products);
- Substance abuse (reduce or eliminate intake; abstain altogether);
- Medications (take a new one, take a different one, stop taking one, replace one with another, take at a different time); and
- Glucose (monitor levels in the blood, ingest more/less liquid).

Rollnick et al. also suggest recruiting a team of practitioners to address the patient's health problem(s). These include physicians, nurses, dieticians, exercise coaches, physical therapists, dental practitioners, and mental health professionals.

Determine Sources of Client Motivation to Enhance Commitment

Health behavior change cannot occur without the client's full commitment. Clients must have a motive to reduce or eliminate habits that they "know" are unhealthy or in some way undesirable and to replace them with habits that are perceived by the client as beneficial, either in the short term, long term, or both. This is why the DVM includes a component that asks the client to indicate the "benefits," "costs," and "long-term consequences" of a current unhealthy habit. This process is especially important and effective if the client, rather than the mental health professional or coach, generate this information.

Clients may be asked this question: "On a scale of 1 (very low commitment level) to 10 (very high commitment level), how committed are you to changing your behavior and replacing the unhealthy habit with a better, more desirable one?" If the client answers any number less than 10, the professional must ask the client to explain the gap between the optimal commitment level—10—and the number (less than 10) he or she provided. Often, it seems that clients explain the number they provide as due to a lack the confidence in being able to achieve the goal of changing habits. Clearly some issues, such as the source(s) of low confidence and any other reasons for lower-than-desirable commitment level, have to be discussed, as well as any part of the action plan that completes the model. Clients must be fully committed to changing at least one undesirable habit and also be committed to becoming realigned with their deepest values.

References

Corbin, C. B., & Lindsey, R. (1994). *Concepts of physical fitness with laboratories* (8th ed.). Dubuque, IA: W.C. Brown & Benchmark Publishers.

Hagger, M.S., & Chatzisarantis, N.L.D. (Eds.). *Intrinsic motivation and self-determination in exercise and sport*. Champaign, IL: Human Kinetics.

Hellston, L.A. M., & Rogers, W.T. (2009). Development and preliminary validation of the Time Management for Exercise Scale. *Measurement in Physical Education and Exercise Science, 13*, 13–33.

Howley, E.T., & Franks, B.D. (2007). *Fitness professional's handbook* (5th ed.). Champaign, IL: Human Kinetics.

Lox, C.L., Martin Ginis, K.A., & Petruzzello, S.J. ((2014). *The psychology of exercise* (4th ed.). Scottsdale, AZ: Holcomb Hathaway.

Martin Ginis, K.A., Burke, S.M., & Gauvin, L. (2007). Exercising with others exacerbates the negative effects of mirrored environments on sedentary women's feeling states. *Psychology and Health, 22*, 945–962.

Maslach, C., & Jackson, S.E. (1981). The measurement of experienced burnout. *Journal of Organizational Behavior, 2*, 99–113.

O'Rourke, M. (2011). *Predictors of attitudes toward physical activity as a function of secondary school physical education experiences among adults*. A doctoral dissertation at Middle Tennessee State University, Murfreesboro, TN.

Rollnick, S., Mason, P., Butler, C. (1999). *Health behavior change: A guide for practitioners*. New York: Churchill Livingstone.

Sallis, J.F., & Owen, N. (1999). *Physical activity & behavioral medicine*. Thousand Oaks, CA: Sage.

Vansteenkiste, M., Soenens, B., & Lens, W. (2007). Intrinsic versus extrinsic goal promotion in exercise and sport: Understanding the differential impacts on performance and persistence. In M.S. Hagger & N.L.D. Chatzisarantis (Eds.), *Intrinsic motivation and self-determination in exercise and sport* (pp. 167–180). Champaign, IL: Human Kinetics.

PART II

Theoretical Foundations and Support

3

PSYCHOLOGICAL BENEFITS OF PHYSICAL ACTIVITY

Because exercise and other forms of physical activity are often neglected by so many individuals, it is important to address the psychological benefits of an active lifestyle. As the literature indicates, exercise can slow the aging process and improve memory and other forms of cognition (information processing). This is especially relevant for mental health professionals who should be incorporating exercise as part of their client therapy intervention plans.

Results of past published studies have consistently revealed that exercise has highly favorable effects on mental health and well-being. Aerobic exercise (cardiovascular; high heart rate), in particular, strongly influences various areas of mental health and numerous psychological factors. Perhaps the most notable changes in psychological functioning concern stress, anxiety, mood, self-esteem, and depression. When applying the DVM, therapists and coaches will want to pay special attention to making physical activity a primary component of a client's/patient's action plan, which is the model's last segment.

Positive Stress

Several studies have confirmed that exercise—both acute (i.e., short term; one day or a single exercise bout) and chronic (i.e., long term; weeks, months, and years)—markedly reduces negative forms of stress and increases what might be called "positive stress." Positive stress includes anything that causes energy to be expended physically, mentally, emotionally, and spiritually. Positive stress provides the energy needed for growth, improvement, and development. In addition, stress-related problems can be reduced, even eliminated, by what is called "voluntary recovery" from life's demands and storms. Recovery allows us to renew "or recapture" our energy. Weight training, which has an anabolic (body-tissue building) effect on the human system, and other forms of physical activity are examples of positive stress (see Anshel, 2012 and Loehr, 1997, for further explanations of the concepts of positive stress and recovery).

It is thought that reduced stress and other psychological benefits of exercise or other forms of physical activity can be explained by the *distraction hypothesis*, in which the exerciser is concentrating on the exercise activity and avoiding or reducing stressful thoughts. The combination of pleasant thoughts also increase feelings of self-control; the lack of self-control is a source of acute and chronic stress.

The two important caveats of the stress-reducing effects of exercise is that the person must *enjoy* exercising or any other form of vigorous physical activity (e.g., skiing, bicycling, sport participation) and that the activity session be a minimum of 30 minutes. It is also highly desirable, though not mandatory, that the activity be aerobic (increased heart rate), as opposed to various forms of nonaerobic exercise (e.g., resistance training); however, yoga and Pilates also have stress-reducing effects. Finally, aerobic exercise programs should last at least a few months for reducing chronic stress.

At the same time, it is important to mention that exercising will not reduce stress and, in fact, may *increase* stress if the individual is required or coerced into exercising, such as exercising for punishment in school PE or on sports teams. Therefore, it is essential that the person engage in the type of exercise he or she enjoys, it is not too strenuous, and it is convenient in terms of exercise location and times of the day and week. A forced exercise location, type, and time will only lead to dropping out. Human tissue improves its efficiency in response to exercise and other forms of physical activity. We become stronger and more resilient to life's storms.

State Anxiety

Anxiety, which is a condition that differs from stress, consists of feelings of worry or threat. Stress reflects a person's perception of *immediate* danger or a physiological response related to confrontation or escape, often termed "fight or flight response." Anxiety, often referred to as *state anxiety*, on the other hand, reflects an individual's current (situational) perceptions of *future* harm. Students often feel anxiety prior to taking a school examination, for example, due to feelings of worry about not performing well. An overweight person might feel self-conscious and anxious about his or her appearance or poor exercise performance while engaging in a group exercise class. It is not uncommon for individuals to perform poorly when experiencing state anxiety due, in part, to muscular tension—called somatic anxiety—and/or poor psychological functioning—called cognitive anxiety.

Anxiety can also be part of a person's disposition; people can feel anxious as part of their personality. Trait anxiety is stable across situations and is not amenable to change; it can be measured with a written inventory. A person with high trait anxiety is predisposed to perceive apparently harmless situations as threatening. Exercise will not change his or her trait anxiety level, but it can alter his or her disposition to feel anxiety in a certain situation, a condition called state anxiety. A low trait anxious individual is less susceptible to situational anxiety than a high trait anxious person. In summary, state anxiety, but not trait anxiety, may reduce stress when performing various forms of physical activity perceived by the individual as pleasant, thereby distracting the person from stressful thoughts. Aerobic exercise has also benefited patients with various anxiety disorders (e.g., panic disorder, post-traumatic stress disorder) and clinical depression (Petruzzello et al., 1991).

Mood

Mood, often called "mood state," is a situational characteristic, ranging from immediate to one week in duration. Because mood is usually measured as a state (situational), not trait, characteristic, research on the effects of exercise on mood have focused on immediate, rather than long-term, effects. In their comprehensive review of the research literature spanning 25 years related to the effects of exercise on mood, Berger and Motl (2000) found conclusive evidence for mood-enhancing effects of exercise. These studies used the Profile of Mood States, showing improved vigor and reduced tension, depression, anger, confusion, and fatigue within one week of an exercise session. The authors attributed changes in mood following exercise to *psychological mechanisms*, including "enhanced self-concept, feelings of self-efficacy, enjoyment, expectancy of psychological benefits, 'time out' from one's routine and daily hassles, and an increased sense of control" (p. 84). The authors recommend that unless a participant prefers low or high exercise intensity, optimal conditions for mood changes occur at a moderate intensity level.

Reasons for Mood Changes from Exercise

There are several possible explanations for experiencing an elevated positive mood state following exercise or, for that matter, following most forms of physical activity.

Distraction/time-out hypothesis. Because exercise has stress-reducing properties, it distracts the individual from stressful and negative thoughts and feelings, thereby improving mood. Stress, anxiety, and negative feelings are either forgotten or ignored while the person's attentional focus is on the exercise task, the environment in which exercise is performed, or toward individuals who form an integral part of the exercise experience. Exercise is an excellent "time out" strategy from the day's demands.

Thermogenic hypothesis. Another explanation for a positive mood following exercise is that the elevation of body temperature due to exercise has a relaxing effect. Researchers have found that elevating body temperature produces a therapeutic benefit, such as muscle relaxation. It is thought that a similar reaction follows exercise, which results in an elevated internal body temperature. A similar change in psychological factors may occur, such as reduced anxiety and other negative feelings.

Social interaction hypothesis. Exercise may improve mood state if the individual exercises in the company of others, which is a common reaction, and enjoys this type of environment. This is especially true in special programs that improve health, fitness, or rehabilitation and consists of a group of individuals who meet regularly to experience therapy, such as patients who attend postcoronary exercise programs.

The social interaction hypothesis also explains the value of a related concept called *social support.* The results of numerous studies clearly indicate that individuals who exercise with others—a form of *direct* social support—or receive verbal encouragement from others—a form of *indirect* social support—are more likely to have positive feelings about their exercise program and maintain their participation, as opposed to persons who want to exercise with others but, instead, do so alone.

Endorphin hypothesis. Another possible cause of mood change following exercise is a function of biochemical changes, called endorphins, due to exercise activity. Exercise is performed to excess due to the person's dependence, sometimes called an addiction, on the release of endorphins during exercise. This process is thought to at least partially explain exercise dependence in which the person is literally addicted to exercise, especially cardiovascular exercise. Optimal conditions for mood changes for all of these possible explanations occur at a *moderate* intensity level.

Self-Esteem

Self-esteem, also referred to as self-worth, concerns the degree to which individuals value or approve of their identity (i.e., how the person feels about who he or she is). Self-esteem is a multidimensional concept, meaning that it includes different sources. Positive self-esteem is associated with good mental health.

Dimensions of self-esteem include knowledge (academic), physical/somatic, sport, social, religious, family, and work. Exercise is more likely to improve self-esteem if the individual considers exercise enjoyable; if the person feels a sense of achievement due to improving his or her exercise performance and fitness; and if exercise is related to good health and, in the exerciser's eyes, improved physical appearance (e.g., avoiding obesity, maintaining proper body weight).

Whether exercise improves self-esteem is related to the person's initial level of self-esteem. Positive associations between exercise and self-esteem have been found, but effects are stronger for individuals initially lower in self-esteem. In addition, exercise has more potent effects on physical self-concept and self-esteem than on general self-perceptions. Among females, exercise improves self-esteem, especially if the individual is comfortable and secure with her physical characteristics and appearance, often called body or physique self-esteem. That is, in relation to physical activity, individuals link their self-worth—their sense of value and competence—to their physical attributes. Concomitant changes in other forms of self-esteem (e.g., family, academic, sport) were not noted.

Cognitive Functioning

Cognitive functioning describes how we process information so that we can learn meaningful information and perform motor skills. It is helpful to describe a brief overview of the information processing sequence. While researchers still debate the most accurate depiction of how we learn and perform motor skills, most models of this literature include the following content and sequence.

Information processing begins by a process called *stimulus detection,* that is, identifying one or more stimuli in the environment that can either be ignored or receive attention. In the second stage, either a single stimulus or many stimuli selectively pass through a "filter" mechanism that separates meaningful from non-meaningful content. Stimuli that pass through the filter are *perceived, categorized,* or *interpreted.* This stage is called *perception;* the person attempts to make sense out of the stimulus.

In the next stage, called *short-term memory,* the information is internally rehearsed with a process called *covert rehearsal.* Thus, after information is perceived, it is either rehearsed (i.e., thinking/reflecting) or immediately used then often forgotten. In short-term memory, the person typically reacts quickly to the stimulus and does not store it. The short-term memory mechanism allows for information to be stored for later recall if stored into *long-term (permanent) memory.*

Whether the person makes a rapid decision or stores the information often depends on how much time is needed to complete the task or how quickly they must react. Not all tasks and skills require rehearsal; sometimes a rapid response void of thinking time is needed. React or don't react. Forgetfulness that accompanies a concussion or dementia is usually located in short-term memory. If a rapid, often coordinated response is needed, the person executes the skill generated by a mechanism called the *motor program*—a series of coordinated and timed movements that result in meaningful performance.

Finally, most meaningful movements and performance outcomes are accompanied by two forms of feedback, internal (i.e., kinesthetic, or tactual information) and external (visual and auditory input). Cognitive functioning, then, is defined as the process of taking in/detecting, perceiving/interpreting, storing/remembering, determining/deciding, and responding to/executing an action at the proper speed, accuracy, and efficiency. The important point about cognitive functioning in the present context is that exercise, especially aerobic (cardiovascular) exercise (as opposed to flexibility and strength training), improves the speed, efficiency, and accuracy of cognitive functioning.

Exercise, particularly of an aerobic (high heart rate) nature, improves cognitive functioning in the areas of attentional focusing, concentration, monitoring one's thought processes and emotions, storing and retrieving information, and performing motor skills. The aging process normally slows and reduces the capability of the brain and nervous system to function at optimal levels. The combination of aging and a sedentary lifestyle expedites the effects of aging on cognitive functioning.

Exercise reverses the effects of aging on cognitive functioning. In their extensive review of this literature, Lox, Martin Ginis, and Petruzzello (2014) concluded that regular exercise results in improvements in cognitive function and even reverses the loss of function seen with aging. Does a single exercise bout, however, benefit cognitive functioning? Using laboratory tasks, such as reaction time (i.e., the time interval between detecting a stimulus and initiating a response), decision-making speed, and visual tracking, Lox et al. concluded that even a single bout of activity may have short-term benefits in terms of enhancing information-processing capacity. It appears, therefore, that exercise has both short-term and long-term benefits in cognitive functioning.

Depression

Depression falls under a category of mental disorders, as listed in *The Mental Health Desk Reference* (Welfel & Ingersoll, 2001). The manual classifies depression as a mood disturbance that includes disorders that influence mood regulation. Exercise has been shown to reduce symptoms of depression. Its characteristics include sustained feelings of sadness or elation, feelings of guilt or worthlessness, disturbances in appetite, disturbances in sleep patterns, lack of energy, difficulty concentrating, loss of interest in all or most activities, problems with memory, thoughts of suicide, and hallucinations

Depression research has taken primarily two forms: exercise as a *preventive* measure of depression and effects of exercise on *existing* depression. Extensive reviews of literature by Fox et al. (2014) and Biddle and Mutrie (2001) have shown extensive benefits of exercise on both depression prevention and remedy. These reviews clearly indicate that sedentary, inactive adult females were twice as likely to develop depression as compared to moderately active women. In addition, there is an association between inactivity and incidence of depression. The risk of developing depression is significantly greater for both men and women if they do not engage in regular exercise. In addition, physical activity at baseline is negatively associated with depression in later life, whereas more activity early in life predicts lower subsequent depression.

Can exercise serve as a treatment for depression? Absolutely. In a meta-analysis of 80 studies, North et al. (1990) found that exercise: (a) resulted in decreased depression, (b) was as or more effective than traditional therapies, and (c) that all types of exercise (e.g., weight training, cardiovascular, yoga) resulted in reduced depression. Weight training, aerobic activity, and walking each reduced depression for both men and women. The optimal conditions under which exercise will improve clinical depression occurred when exercise training lasts at least five weeks, is performed at least three times per week, is of low to moderate intensity level (50% of predicted maximum heart rate), and that each bout was at least 20 to 60 minutes in duration.

In summary, physical activity, in general, and formal exercise (e.g., jogging, brisk walking, resistance training), in particular, will favorably influence various components of psychological characteristics. These include mood, cognitive functioning, including the concomitant aging effects in relation to processing information, anxiety, and depression. The most important aspect of these benefits, however, is consistency in developing a long-term exercise habit. These positive outcomes are not likely to occur when exercise is haphazard, inconsistent, uses little exertion (e.g., taking a slow stroll), and is forced (i.e., the individual does not enjoy the experience or is asked to perform an activity that is not pleasant).

References

Anshel, M.H. (2012). *Sport psychology: From theory to practice* (5th ed.). San Francisco: Benjamin-Cummings.

Berger, B. G., & Motl, R.W. (2000). Exercise and mood: A selective review and synthesis of research employing the Profile of Mood States. *Journal of Applied Sport Psychology, 12*, 69–92.

Biddle, S.J.H., & Mutrie, N. (2001). Depression and other mental illnesses. In S.J.H. Biddle & N. Mutrie (Eds.), *Psychology of physical activity: Determinants, well-being and interventions* (pp. 202–235). London: Routledge.

Loehr, J. (1997). *Stress for success*. New York: Three Rivers Press.

Lox, C.L., Martin Ginis, K.A., & Petruzzello, S.J. (2014). *The psychology of exercise: Integrating theory and practice*. Scottsdale, AZ: Holcomb Hathaway.

North, T.C., McCullagh, P., & Tran, Z.V. (1990). Effect of exercise on depression. *Exercise & Sport Sciences Reviews, 18*, 379–415.

Petruzzello, S.J., Landers, D.M., Hatfield, B., Kubitz, K.A., Salazar, W. (1991). A meta- analysis on the anxiety-reducing effects of acute and chronic exercise: Outcomes and mechanisms. *Sports Medicine, 11*, 143–182.

Welfel, E.R., & Ingersoll, R.E. (2001). *The mental health desk reference: A practice-based guide to diagnosis, treatment, and professional ethics*. New York: John C. Wiley & Sons.

4

STRENGTHS AND LIMITATIONS OF EXISTING THEORIES AND MODELS IN HEALTH BEHAVIOR CHANGE

It is well known that people often do not consider the health consequences for their actions. As indicated earlier, changing unhealthy habits is enormously challenging for most individuals. The primary objective of the DVM is to replace our self-destructive habits with more desirable and healthier one's. The model helps clients/patients to voluntarily engage in health behavior change for the purpose of preventing illness, improving general health, managing disease to receive a better diagnosis, and receiving treatment, or rehabilitation, in restoring health or reducing disease progression (e.g., Clark & Becker, 1998; Ockene, 2001).

To determine which interventions are most effective at improving health behavior, researchers and practitioners need to examine their efficacy. Most of the existing published intervention research has been guided by various theories and models that explain and predict improved health outcomes. Personal, environmental, and situational factors each influence these outcomes. The primary purpose of theories and models is to explain, describe, or predict behavior in the attempt to advance knowledge. It is wrong to think that theories and models have minimal value in applied settings. Let's review the concepts of theories and models.

What Is a Theory?

A *theory* is usually defined as a set of general principles that attempts to explain and predict a person's thoughts, emotions, and behavior, often by combining environmental (e.g., exercising in a fitness club as opposed to alone at home), situational (e.g., performance under competitive versus noncompetitive conditions), and personal factors (e.g., a person's level of self-confidence or level of skill or fitness). Predicting behavior is a very powerful tool in trying to understand how to promote or increase some actions, while inhibiting or eliminating others. How, for instance, can we improve the likelihood of a person's need to follow a particular eating pattern, use mental skills for reducing stress, or initiate a new exercise program as well as predict the optimal conditions for adhering to the program? The value of theories is to help answers those types of questions. The key element of a theory is the intention to *predict* future behavior.

While the intention of a theory is to predict certain outcomes, a *model*, on the other hand, is a visual representation of the combination of thoughts, attitudes, emotions, and behaviors that reflect a series of structures (i.e., the "boxes" in the model's figure), each connected by one or more processes (i.e., the "arrows" that connect two or more structures), that eventually lead to a predetermined outcome. The structures are stable and permanent, while the processes are changeable and may be influenced by interventions such as using mental skills or changing thought content. For example, a model might illustrate that an individual's self-talk content—positive or negative—influences attitudes toward exercise, emotional content (e.g., perceived effort, mood state, anxiety level) during exercise, and/or the level of exercise performance. The research question in this example would be whether self-talk content, both prior to and during a specific exercise period, influences the person's attitude toward exercise and the individual's exercise intensity and endurance.

In summary, theories and models are needed: (a) to improve our understanding of the interrelationships between a person's thoughts (also called *cognitions*), emotions (also called *affect*), and behaviors (or performance); (b) to help explain behavioral phenomena, that is, why certain actions occur under particular circumstances, (c) to predict future behavior, (d) to simplify complex and abundant information into a coherent and organized structure that improves our understanding of these processes, and (e) to test the effectiveness of interventions, often as part of research, that can improve certain predetermined outcomes.

Numerous theories have been proposed over the years that relate to predicting and explaining health-related behaviors. These theories and models have been met with *limited* success in promoting health behavior change, with relatively low prediction for exercise behavior. For example, one limitation of most theories and models of health behavior change has been the assumption that participants in a study *want to* change their behavior. This is incorrect. Still, many of these models are still being tested and, in some cases, partially supported. Here is a brief review of selected and well-published theories and models.

Health Belief Model (HBM)

The HBM (Becker & Maiman, 1975) posits that most people adopt habits based on what is in their best interests, including good health. Actions will not occur, on the other hand, if people believe they will lead to unhealthy outcomes. Thus, if people feel that engaging in regular exercise will improve health and have other advantages, they will more likely begin and in some cases maintain an exercise habit.

HBM predicts people's healthy habits if they are concerned about or are currently experiencing poor health, feeling susceptible to health problems, and feeling empowered to prevent or control health problems. Thus, individuals make decisions that affect their health either to start or to stop actions that are in their best interest, such as tobacco use. Decisions about changing health behavior are predicated on establishing a balance between the individual's perceptions of the level of seriousness of one's condition versus the likelihood that behavior change will reduce the threat to one's health.

Perhaps one immediate limitation of the HBM is that the consequences of unhealthy habits often take many years to experience; there is no immediate threat to one's health and well-being. People, however, are far more likely to change unhealthy behavior(s) if they receive a serious, life-threatening diagnosis from a medical practitioner or experience a life-threatening event, and their medical practitioner recommends specific changes to their current lifestyle. Thus, in support of the HBM, initiating a new, healthier habit is far more likely when there is a sense of urgency about one's current health status—ostensibly due to a particular, clearly identified health problem—and the perception that the problem will be remedied by adopting a new habit or lifestyle. Oldridge and Streiner (1990) found that predicting a person's readiness to exercise was most predictive if exercise was perceived as effective and improved general health.

HBM has several limitations, one of which is that the HBM can predict exercise participation only to the extent that an individual links exercise habits with improved health. For individuals who do not perceive their health is at risk, however, the HBM is less effective at predicting future health and exercise behavior. Adolescents and young adult males, for example, are particularly known to engage more frequently in high-risk behaviors, such as using tobacco products, mind-altering drugs, and alcohol. They drive faster than the rest of the population as well. The HBM, therefore, does not seem as powerful in predicting health behaviors of relatively young individuals, as opposed to middle-aged and older groups.

Another limitation of the HBM is that it is based on initiating and explaining behavior rather than explaining and predicting healthy habits. The HBM is more useful for *preventive* health behaviors and compliance with medical regimens, but it is much weaker when it is applied to developing an exercise habit. A final limitation of the HBM is that it does not suggest intervention strategies that develop and maintain healthy habits. Who will adhere versus discontinue the new healthy habit? The HBM does not address this question.

Theories of Reasoned Action and Planned Behavior

The theory of planned behavior (TPB) is an extension and modification of the theory of reasoned action (TRA; Ajzen & Fishbein, 1974). Both theories attempt to determine and predict the factors that influence an individual's actions in social settings. To Ajzen and Fishbein, people's actions reflect their beliefs about the appropriateness of their actions, the outcome they expect from their actions, and the importance they place on these outcomes. At the center of TRA in predicting health behaviors are three components: the person's *attitudes* about the behavior ("I enjoy exercising because. . . ."; (2) the *social norms* of that behavior, that is, its acceptability and commonality among friends and the surrounding culture; and (3) the person's *intentions* to perform the health behaviors (e.g., "I intend to take a brisk walk nightly after coming home from work"; "I will not have a full meal within two hours of bedtime"). Attitudes toward any habit perceived as "healthy" reflect the person's beliefs about the habit's benefits, as opposed to its costs or long-term undesirable consequences.

The second component of TRA consists of subjective social norms about the behavior, specifically, the individual's perceptions about the importance that *others* place on the behavior and the person's incentive to meet their—the others'—expectations. Thus, a person who interacts with family or friends who successfully manage their stress, sleep well, or take the stairs instead of elevators is more likely to adopt these same habits than an individual whose friends and family do not possess these habits or have unfavorable attitudes toward these actions. A healthy habit is more easily attainable if people surround themselves with others who support these habits. As Ajzen and Fishbein (1974) conclude, sometimes *attitude* is the primary predictor of intentions, while other times it is the *social norms* component.

In his modified follow up of TRA, Ajzen (1985) suggested a third component that predicts healthy habits, *perceived behavioral control.* Ajzen contends that it is important that people conclude that they have the personal resources (i.e., skills, motivation, and perseverance) and the opportunity to perform the health behavior or to attain the goal. Thus, individuals with realistic expectations about the likelihood of achieving health behavior change will feel a high degree of control toward reaching their destiny and will more likely feel motivated and committed to achieving health-related goals. Unmet expectations, on the other hand, will lead to disappointment and feelings of low self-control about their apparent inability to meet their health-related goals, such as better sleep, less stress, more exercise, and so on.

In a meta-analysis to determine the extent to which TRA and TPB successfully predicted exercise behavior, Hausenblas, Carron, and Mack (1997) concluded that attitude strongly influences intention to exercise and that intention to exercise predicts exercise behavior. To Hausenblas et al. (1997), "individuals have the greatest commitment to exercise when they hold favorable beliefs about exercise and believe that they can successfully perform the behavior" (p. 45).

There are numerous imitations to TPB and TRA. For instance, a person may believe that a particular habit or behavior pattern is needed for various benefits, yet the same person can offer several excuses for not wanting to engage in the new habit. For instance, the *intention* to exercise does not account for all exercise behavior (Mackinnon, Ritchie, Hooper, & Abernethy, 2003). A person can express the intention to exercise but fail to carry out that intended action.

It is apparent that the components of TRA and TPB-attitude and subjective norm, the person's intention to carry out a new healthy habit, perceived behavioral control—do not necessarily predict health behavior change. A favorable attitude toward the new habit must first be developed before a person adopts it. Identifying the *benefits* of adopting a new and healthy habit in contrast to the *costs* of not adopting the new habit will help promote a desirable attitude to initiate and maintain the new habit. A final limitation is that TRA and TPB offer no *behavioral* interventions that promote starting and sustaining an exercise program.

Self-Efficacy Theory

How confident are you when performing a difficult skill, especially for the first time or in the presence of others? Might you be nervous if your performance is being evaluated? Your level of self-efficacy can influence or even determine your performance success. Self-efficacy is defined as a set of beliefs and expectations about how capable a person feels in performing certain, highly specific behaviors that will lead to achieving desirable outcomes in particular situations (Bandura, 1997). A person can feel high self-efficacy about exercising at a high intensity or demonstrate competence in performing a sport skill yet feel low self-efficacy when it comes to exercising or performing a skill in competitive situations.

In relation to starting a healthier lifestyle, high self-efficacy usually leads to maintaining it as well. Low self-efficacy often predicts quitting the new (healthier) behavior. Perhaps the "good news" is that self-efficacy is task-specific and is not usually generalized to other tasks or under other conditions. Thus, people who believe they are capable of performing "successfully" and meeting their goals will more likely engage in and maintain those actions that are specific to the activity. Expectations of future success and failure strongly influence the person's selection of those activities, the degree of effort expended on the activity, and the degree of adherence to the activity. This is particularly true if peoples' experiences are disappointing, such as not noticing improved fitness or weight loss, for instance.

McAuley and Mihalko (1998) reviewed over 100 studies on the effects of self-efficacy theory on exercise behavior. They concluded that self-efficacy predicts exercise participation and maintenance better under each of four other personal characteristics: perceived choice (of the type of exercise performed); thought patterns, optimal effort, and reasonably high self-expectations.

First, people select the type of exercise behavior undertaken, a process called *perceived choice*. Self-efficacy remains low to moderate if the person did not select the activity to perform; the decision to exercise cannot be forced. Second, people possess certain *thought patterns* that heighten their arousal and level of excitement (e.g., optimism, positive self-talk, intrinsic motivation, feelings of competence and enjoyment). Third, *optimal effort* is needed to meet performance goals. Efforts to overcome barriers and challenges must be redoubled. Finally, people must have *reasonably high expectations* of successful performance and outcomes. To McAuley and Mihalko, the strongest influence of self-efficacy on exercise behavior is *performance accomplishments*, that is, mastering tasks that the people view as challenging.

Self-efficacy theory is not without weaknesses. McAuley and Mihalko claim, for instance, that even with high self-efficacy beliefs, at least concerning exercise, "the decision to embark on an exercise program . . . is fraught with challenges especially when individuals are sedentary, older, or recovering from a life-threatening disease" (p. 372). Engaging in physical activity at the "correct" level of exertion, duration, and frequency to obtain sufficient health and medical benefits is often too unpleasant for many individuals, particularly given the widespread sedentary lifestyle of many individuals. Thus, the "benefits" of remaining sedentary and not exercising (e.g., having more time to do other things, not experiencing the discomfort associated with vigorous exercise) are often greater than the consequences of a sedentary lifestyle. Still, self-efficacy theory often predicts a person's decision to engage—or not engage—in a given task, program, or lifestyle (Bandura, 1997).

Transtheoretical Model

The transtheoretical model (Prochaska & DiClemente, 1983), also called "Stages of Change Model," was originally intended for persons with addictive behaviors. It was later modified by Prochaska and Marcus (1994) to describe stages related to exercise. The model, which is cyclical (i.e., stages can be repeated) and not linear (i.e., continuous), posits that the decision to begin and sustain an exercise habit is a long-term process. The decision to change unhealthy behavior is not always permanent. Each of the model's five stages are briefly described with respect to exercise performance.

Precontemplation. For the first six months, the sedentary individual has no intention of exercising. Common reasons include no perceived "need" to exercise; unpleasant experiences with previous attempts at exercising; lack of social support from significant others to engage in regular exercise; self-consciousness about exercising in a public facility in the presence of fitter, younger, thinner individuals; unable to afford exercise equipment, clothing, or fitness club memberships; or living too far away from available programs and facilities.

Contemplation. The person now *intends* to start a regular exercise habit, usually within the next six months. Often, the individual has learned about the advantages of exercise through written materials; advice from a physician; or at the urging of friends, family members, a health professional, or sports coach. Exercise testing, prescription, and/or coaching may come from their health care provider. Another exercise objective is to maintain a "better" appearance through improved musculature and reduced body weight and fat. The individual now believes that the "costs" of not exercising are becoming excessive and damaging, while the benefits are increasingly more attractive. Prochaska and Marcus (1994) report that "on the average, individuals stay in this relatively stable stage for at least 2 years, telling themselves that someday they will change but putting off change" (p. 162). These individuals are called *chronic contemplators*.

Preparation. The person is now more serious about an exercise program and *intends* to start exercising "in the near future," usually within a month. Often, an action plan is formulated, usually by a fitness coach who has the expertise to prescribe and monitor the exerciser's progress and provide high-quality instruction. It is important that the plan obtain the optimal benefits (e.g., exercising only once per week rather than at least three times a week, not exercising at sufficient intensity, performing strength training but ignoring aerobic work). The individual is not yet fully committed to the plan because the perceived barriers to exercise (e.g., not enough time, physical discomfort due to exertion, cost of a fitness club membership or purchasing equipment, lack of time) still outweigh the benefits.

Action. The person has initiated and maintained an exercise routine for under six months. Dropping out of the exercise program and reverting to an inactive lifestyle (called "relapsing") is still very possible. One uncertainty about this stage concerns the criteria that constitute "action." This stage-action-is defined operationally (i.e., each situation determines the criteria for "action"). This is important, not only to experience the desirable outcomes of an exercise plan but to determine if exercisers are adhering to the program. Have they maintained participation at the proper level or are they only partially complying? As Prochaska and Marcus (1994) conclude, "problems exist in areas for which there is no agreed upon criteria" (p. 163).

Maintenance. After a period of six months, there is now less likelihood that the person will quit the exercise program. There is uncertainty in the literature, however, about the operational definition of "maintenance," not unlike uncertainty about how the action stage is defined. Rand and Weeks (1998) have generated various terms and concepts that help clarify various categories of maintenance that reflect a person's intended and planned exercise behavior. Examples include "partial adherence," "ideal adherence," "appropriate adherence," "erratic adherence," and "involuntary adherence" to reflect the criterion of "maintenance" (i.e., adherence). Thus, exercising once per week instead of the planned or prescribed three times per week reflects *partial* adherence, or not exercising due to injury is an example of *involuntary* adherence. Prochaska and Marcus (1992) claim that an exercise period of at least five years is the likely criterion for establishing a *permanent* exercise habit and not return to their previous nonexercise lifestyle.

Termination. The person feels 100% confident that he or she will not return to their former inactive lifestyle that neglected an exercise habit. Still, reverting to previous habits, including the absence of regular exercise, remains possible. Why? Because exercise barriers do not go away. The same perceived barriers exist at this stage that prevented exercising in the first place. As indicated earlier, these barriers include *perceived* excessive demands on one's time, experiencing pain or injury, experiencing one or more unpleasant exercise-related situations (e.g., exercising for punishment), poor weather, breakage of equipment, more tempting activities that replace exercise, the absence of others' encouragement (e.g., lack of social support), failure to meet goals, increased exercise difficulty due to weight gain or aging, and lack of financial resources to afford a fitness club membership or afford to purchase exercise clothing/equipment.

Perhaps not surprisingly, there are limitations to the transtheoretical (stages of change) model. For example, Bandura (1997) claims the model fails to reflect fundamental tenets of the traditional stage theory of a natural progression in which one stage is operationally linked to each succeeding stage. This is not the case here. In addition, Rosen's (2000) meta-analysis indicated that readiness for exercise may not be a discrete (i.e., yes-no) variable but a continuous variable (i.e., not at all-very little-somewhat-very much-extremely). In addition, to test the model's efficacy requires providing individuals with intervention strategies that are compatible with their particular exercise stage and then measuring their exercise behavior over a prolonged period of time, perhaps several years. And, as noted earlier, selected stages (e.g., action) need to be operationally defined. What is one form of "action" for one study may differ for another study.

Relapse Prevention Model

The relapse prevention model (Marlatt & Gordon, 1985) reflects self-controlled (self-regulation) efforts for maintaining desirable behaviors, such as exercise, and to resist feelings and situations that promote reverting back to former, undesirable behavior patterns. With respect to exercise, the person is taught to use cognitive (e.g., positive self-talk, visualization) and behavioral strategies (e.g., music, goal-setting, social support, record keeping) to deal productively with exercise relapses.

High-risk situations, such as feeling uncomfortable entering a fitness facility, not knowing how to use exercise equipment, being injured or ill, or experiencing pain during early attempts in starting an exercise program, often initiate the relapse process. Situations that challenge a person's confidence in his or her ability to meet exercise goals or that lack social support (i.e., social support) also promote relapse.

One negative condition that predicts relapse is called the *abstinence violation effect* (Lox et al., 2014). This condition occurs when the person quits his or her exercise habit after missing several exercise sessions, perhaps due to illness, injury, or some other reasons beyond his or her control. The person may feel hopeless in the quest to reach a particular goal in establishing the new (healthy) habit rather than being patient with regaining control of the situation and reestablishing the habit.

The abstinence violation effect reflects "all or none" thinking. The individual views his or her participation as either full adherence to the new habit or failing to maintain the habit at all. There is no gray area. To make matters worse, the person considers him/herself a failure in taking responsibility for reaching goals and establishing the new habit and, eventually, a lifestyle change. The relapse prevention model is intuitively appealing in promoting exercise behavior and adherence. Exercise relapse, however, is clearly a significant problem, and any approach to minimize this process is needed.

Limitations of the relapse prevention model are that the model was developed to stop high-frequency undesirable behaviors. Exercise, however, is a low-frequency desirable behavior. It is difficult, therefore, to detect an exercise lapse or to deal with a lapse in a timely manner to prevent quitting permanently. In addition, the model does not account for overcoming an adherence violation effect, in which missing one or more exercise sessions permanently abandons future exercise habits. Factors such as lifestyle imbalances and prioritizing self-gratification (e.g., leading a sedentary lifestyle) over devotion and energy toward more health-enhancing activities are not adequately addressed by this model. Thus, while the Relapse Prevention Model provides valuable insights into strategies for promoting exercise adherence, it lacks the incentives and strategies for developing a long-term commitment to exercise.

Self-Determination Theory

Most persons have three primary psycho-social needs, according to Deci and Ryan (1985): to feel self-determining, or autonomous; to demonstrate competence; and to maintain social interaction, or relatedness. Persons are motivated to seek challenges and take risks attempting to satisfy one or more of these needs.

Three types of motivation drive achievement behavior: intrinsic, extrinsic, and amotivation. *Intrinsic motivation* explains a person's desire to perform a task due to feelings of pleasure or satisfaction. *Extrinsic motivation*, on the other hand, drives behavior based on four types of regulation: confirming a sense of self ("I feel better about myself when I exercise"), achieving personal goals (called integrated regulation), feeling required to maintain or to improve health, and gaining a reward or avoiding punishment to prevent social rejection.

Amotivation is the relative absence of motivation or intention to engage in a healthy habit, including the lack of perceived skills, history of starting and then quitting the habit, and feeling the habit is unnecessary or unimportant. Only limited research has supported the validity of the self-determination theory to explain and predict exercise behavior (see Hagger & Chatzisarantis, 2008, for a review). For example, the theory predicts that persons who exercise to improve physical appearance, which is a common exercise motive (i.e., low self-determination), would less likely adhere to their exercise habit than a person who engages in exercise for pleasure (i.e., high self-determination).

The exercise motives of improved physical appearance, superior health, energy, and weight loss are very strong incentives to exercise, irrespective of a sense of satisfaction and enjoyment from exercising. Although high self-determination has been shown to be related to a more positive mood state, further research is needed to examine the influence of self-determination on starting and maintaining healthy habits.

Overview of Limitations of Health Behavior Models and Theories

All theories and models have strengths and limitations. One such limitation associated with each of these theories and models is that researchers need to reach a consensus on the specific behaviors, attitudes, or emotions they want to explain, describe, predict, or change. For example, to address the factors that will promote an exercise habit, researchers and practitioners need to determine if "exercise" is operationally defined as physical activity based on reaching a certain intensity, duration, and frequency or whether any form of physical activity-sport participation or bicycling, for instance-is included in developing an exercise habit.

Most persons will report that they exercise if they "go for a daily walk," however, taking a casual walk will not result in similar physiological and psychological benefits as more vigorous types of exercise. Others will categorize themselves as "exercisers" if they lift weights or engage in yoga or Pilates.

The type of exercise reported in these studies and reviews of literature forms another limitation of most health-related theories and models. For instance, is the theory that predicts behavior addressing a certain behavior pattern or behavior that occurs only under certain conditions or situations? The validity of theories and models in explaining and predicting behavior is clouded by the failure to recognize the unique conditions and situations in which the person's actions occur.

Examining evidence of psychopathology in determining and predicting a person's unhealthy, self-destructive habits is another needed future area of study. For example, clinical (chronic) depression results in reduced energy and the self-motivation to change habits (e.g., starting a new stress management program, diet, or exercise). Chronic anxiety, low self-esteem, irrational thinking, and other psychopathology are strong mediators in predicting and explaining unhealthy behavior. Inclusion of clinical psychology interventions is needed to detect and treat psychopathological conditions that will directly influence attitudes toward behaviors that the person knows are unhealthy and self-destructive.

Implications of Theories and Models for Coaches, Therapists, and Consultants

This section consists of a review of each theory or model with direct implications for consulting clients.

Self-efficacy theory indicates that improving healthy habits by changing health behavior is more likely if clients maintain reasonably high expectations about the positive outcomes that will result from the new habit. In addition, clients should feel they have the skills and perseverance to maintain the new habit, rather than to begin something that will not endure. Therefore, they should receive proper instruction about performing the new habit and techniques for adhering to it. They need to know that changing habits is challenging and requires considerable time and patience.

The client's motivation to exercise, for instance, should improve based on the following types of statements coming from his or her fitness coach: (a) express positive outcome expectations (e.g., "You should be able to do five jog-walk intervals for the next 15 minutes"); (b) confidence in meeting those expectations (e.g., "Your fitness test scores and current body weight and age indicate you should feel confident in completing this task"); and (c) the belief that following a certain exercise regimen will lead to particular (desirable) outcomes, called *efficacy expectations* (e.g., "If you persist on this exercise program, you should be able to lose at least a few pounds by the end of this month"). Consultants need to convincingly and sincerely inform their clients that they—clients—are capable of performing the behaviors that lead to desirable outcomes and these outcomes should be achieved. For example, it is essential that the person engage in the type of exercise he or she enjoys that is not too strenuous and is convenient in terms of exercise location and times of the day and week. "Forcing" or "requiring" novice exercisers to engage in certain—perhaps undesirable—types of exercise at a specific location or at a specific time of day may alienate and demotivate them from developing a favorable attitude toward regular exercise and, eventually, lead to quitting.

These types of demands have formed one important limitation to numerous exercise studies in which a program "dropout" was defined as someone who did not attend a specific group exercise session held at a fitness facility. It was possible, however, that the person decided against exercising at the researcher's mandatory time and place. Another type of exercise intervention that consultants should consider using to improve behaviors related to exercise is called the *self-monitoring checklist*.

Self-Monitoring Checklists

A self-monitoring checklist is not a theory or a model. Its purpose is to provide reminders or guidelines about a person's preparation, thoughts, emotions, or actions (Anshel, 2014). A checklist is like a "to-do" list; instead of predicting, it consists of a list of "reminders" to maintain a particular maintain specific actions until the person develops a set of routines that, with time, become habits.

The term often used in the research literature that refers to following a certain set of mental or physical tasks is called *self-monitoring*. Self-monitoring is a common practice in the diet and nutrition literature in terms of the type, amount, and timing of food intake. Thus, the checklist consists of the list of "things to do," while self-monitoring is the process of following, or monitoring, that "to do" list.

Checklists should be reviewed as often as the individual requires until checklist items become automatic and completed consistently as part of the individual's "regular" (i.e., daily? weekly?) routine.

Fitness coaches may use checklists to prescribe exercise routines, both aerobically (e.g., alternate two minutes of jogging and 30 seconds of walking for six intervals) and resistance training (e.g., "lift 70 pounds for six repetitions, followed by a one-minute rest, then lift another six repetitions, rest for one minute, then lift a final set of six reps"). Fitness coaches may also develop checklists to help individuals prepare for their exercise session; this checklist might include instructions to avoid meals within two hours of aerobic work; maintain proper water intake during the day, during an exercise session, and immediately after an exercise session; and have positive thoughts and self-talk immediately before starting your exercise session.

The self-monitoring checklist was shown to be an effective strategy in one study (Anshel & Seipel, 2009) in which participants—novice exercisers—used the checklist, combined with live coaching, to properly complete a 10-week strength training program, as opposed to the control group that also received coaching but did not use the checklist. See Appendix B for a sample self-monitoring exercise checklist.

References

Ajzen, I. (1985). From intention to actions: A theory of planned behavior. In J. Kuhl and J. Beckman (Eds.), *Action control: From cognition to behavior* (pp. 11–29). Heidelberg: Springer.

Ajzen, I., & Fishbein, M. (1974). Factors influencing intentions and the intention-behavior relation. *Human Relations, 27*, 1–15.

Anshel, M. H., & Seipel, S. J. (2009). Self-monitoring and selected measures of aerobic and strength fitness and short-term exercise adherence. *Journal of Sport Behavior, 32*, 125–151.

Anshel, M.H. (2014). *Applied health fitness psychology*. Champaign, IL: Human Kinetics.

Bandura, A. (1997). *Self-efficacy: The exercise of control.* New York: Freeman.

Becker, M.H., & Maiman, L.A. (1975). Sociobehavioral determinants of compliance with health and medical care recommendations. *Medical Care, 13*, 10–24.

Clark, N.M., & Becker, M.H. (1998). Theoretical models and strategies for improving adherence and disease management. In S.A. Shumaker, E.B. Schron, & W.L. McBee (Eds.), *The handbook of health behavior change* (2nd ed., pp. 5–32).

Deci, E.L., & Ryan, R.M. (1985). *Intrinsic motivation and self-determination in human behavior.* New York: Plenum Press.

Hagger, M.S., & Chatzisarantis, N. (2008). Self-determine theory and the psychology of exercise. International *Journal of Sport and Exercise Psychology, 1*, 79–103.

Hausenblas, H.A., Carron, A.V., & Mack, D.E. (1997). Application of the theories and reasoned action and planned behavior to exercise behavior: A meta-analysis. *Journal of Sport and Exercise Psychology, 19*, 36–51.

Lox, C.L., Martin Ginis, K.A., & Petruzzello, S.J. (2014). *The psychology of exercise: Integrating theory and practice* (4th ed.). Scottsdale, AZ: Holcomb Hathaway.

Mackinnon, L.T., Ritchie, C.B., Hooper, S.L., & Abernethy, P.J. (2003). *Exercise management: Concepts and professional practice*. Champaign, IL: Human Kinetics.

Marlett, G. A., & Gordon, J. R. (1985). *Relapse prevention: Maintenance strategies in addictive behavior change*. New York: Guilford Press.

McAuley, E., & Mihalko, S.L. (1998). Measuring exercise-related self-efficacy. In J.L. Duda (Ed.), *Advances in sport and exercise psychology measurement* (pp.371–381).

Morgantown, WV: Fitness Information, Inc.

Ockene, J.K. (2001). Strategies to increase adherence to treatment. In L.E. Burke & I.S. Ockene (Eds.), *Compliance in healthcare and research* (pp. 43–56). Armonk, NY: Futura.

Oldridge, N.B., & Streiner, D.L. (1990). The health belief model: Predicting compliance and dropout in cardiac rehabilitation. *Medicine and Science in Sports and Exercise, 22*, 678–683.

Prochaska, J. O., & Marcus, B. (1994). The transtheoretical model: Applications to exercise. In R.K. Dishman (Ed.), *Advances in exercise adherence* (pp. 161–180). Champaign, IL: Human Kinetics.

Rand, C. S. & Weeks, K. (1998). Measuring adherence with mediation regimens in clinical care and research. In S. A. Shumaker, E. B. Schron, J. K. Ockene, & W. L. McBee (Eds.), *The handbook of health behavior change* (pp. 114–132). New York: Springer.

Rosen, C. S. (2000). Is the sequencing of change processes by stage consistent across health problems? A meta-analysis. *Health Psychology 19,* 593–604.

5

THEORETICAL AND EMPIRICAL SUPPORT FOR THE DISCONNECTED VALUES MODEL

The DVM is based on strong conceptual and theoretical frameworks and has been empirically tested in applied settings, the results of which have been published in scientific journals. This chapter provides an overview of those studies in order to lend credence to carrying out the model. Thus, the purposes of this chapter are to review existing theoretical cognitive-behavioral frameworks on which the DVM is founded and to provide empirical evidence for the DVM's efficacy. A review of these studies is important to validate the model in applied settings, not only to demonstrate the DVM's strengths but to identify the model's limitations and areas for needed future research.

Conceptual Foundations of the DVM

The DVM is anchored by concepts related to other cognitive-behavioral frameworks that have been successful in changing unhealthy habits. These include cognitive dissonance theory (Festinger, 1957), motivational interviewing (Rollnick, Mason, & Butler, 1999), and acceptance and commitment therapy (Ossman, Wilson, Storaasli, & McNeill (2006). A brief overview and relevance to the present model of each follows.

Cognitive Dissonance Theory

Festinger's (1957) cognitive dissonance theory posits that individuals naturally seek consistency among their cognitions (i.e., beliefs, personal views, emotions, and values). An inconsistency between the person's attitudes (i.e., cognitions) and behaviors results in a state of dissonance and is followed by the people's attempts to change their attitude in order to accommodate these actions. The most important factors that influence the need to change attitude include the number of dissonant beliefs and the importance that people attach to each belief. For example, beliefs about the importance of daily exercise is not be consistent with leading a sedentary lifestyle, not engaging in regular exercise, and being overweight or obese. Dissonance may be minimized or eliminated by one of three strategies: (1) reducing the importance of the conflicting beliefs (e.g., "My whole family is obese; that's the way we are"), (2) acquiring new beliefs that change the balance (e.g., "I am too big and want to live long enough to see my grandchildren grow up"), or (3) removing the conflicting attitude or behavior (e.g., "I will hire a personal trainer to get this body in shape and feel more energy").

Cognitive dissonance theory provides a strong conceptual foundation for the current model in support of the DVM. The DVM, however, goes beyond the recognition of dissonance between values, short-term costs, and long-term consequences of unhealthy habit(s) by including a self-regulation action plan. The plan's purpose is to carry out cognitive-behavior strategies to replace the negative habit with more desirable, healthier routines. Changes in health behavior are more likely if new habits are scheduled and ritualized (Gollwitzer, 1999). The absence of self-regulation action plans has been a weakness in previous exercise adherence programs and studies.

Motivational Interviewing (MI)

The focus of MI is to increase a person's intrinsic motivation (i.e., the sense of task satisfaction, perceived competence, and achievement) for changing his or her health behavior in a favorable way (Rollnick et al., 1999). This is accomplished by collaborating with the client to initiate and maintain desirable changes in behavior, to explore reasons for supporting and not supporting health behavior change, and to help the client take responsibility for behavior change. The client, in consultation with the health professional, determines how and when change will occur.

Rather than relying on teaching clients new mental skills, reshaping thought and emotions, or reexamining the past, MI focuses on current concerns and perspectives. In particular, MI assists clients to make specific changes in their behavior that are most desirable and realistic, while at the same time addressing possible barriers to change. The primary goal of MI is to increase clients' motivation to initiate short-term and long-term behavior change by resolving issues that create ambivalence and resistance. Application of MI techniques has resulted in changes in dietary habits (Resnicow, Jackson, Wang, Dudley, & Baranowski, 2001) and in promoting healthy habits (Resnicow, Dilorio, Soet, Borrelli, Hecht, & Ernst, 2002). Relatively few studies using MI intervention techniques, however, have examined changes in exercise habits.

Acceptance and Commitment Therapy (ACT)

According to Ossman, Wilson, Storaasli, and McNeill (2006), ACT is a form of psychotherapy that addresses a person's tendency to promote and distort unpleasant emotions (e.g., anxiety, anger, guilt), which then lead to engaging in inappropriate behaviors for the intention of avoiding or reducing those unpleasant emotions (e.g., performing risky behaviors, failing to terminate noxious relationships). The goal of ACT is not to change or control undesirable personal and private thoughts or emotions but rather to develop effective behaviors of "proper" daily living to overcome these thoughts or emotions.

ACT consists of clients' willingness to assess their previous attempts at resolving the problem and to determine the success or failure of these attempts. Clients perceive these thoughts as only thoughts, not as truths. There is no conscious attempt to eliminate these unpleasant thoughts. ACT helps clients conclude that accepting their unpleasant emotions leads to a reduction in their intensity or frequency, with acceptance as a strategy designed to reduce or eliminate these undesirable emotions.

Both ACT and the DVM help clients acknowledge "the truth" about their negative (undesirable) habits and their costs and consequences. The clients' goal is not necessarily to eliminate negative habits, which are likely performed daily and ritually. Instead, clients begin process of meeting specific goals or desirable behavior outcomes. In addition, ACT and the DVM help clients to clarify their values and commit to behaviors that are consistent with these values. Finally, ACT and the DVM both require an action plan to experience the benefits of the more desirable habit (e.g., engaging in regular exercise) but without addressing and trying to extinguish all undesirable thoughts or actions. Instead of complete avoidance of the negative habit, the ACT and DVM action plans help the client focus on incorporating new routines.

Review of Empirical Evidence Examining the DVM

The DVM has received empirical support in the extant research literature. Anshel, Brinthaupt, and Kang (2010) and Anshel and Kang (2007), for example, applied the model over a 10-week period with university faculty and staff. Both studies concerned improving exercise habits, as measured by a series of fitness tests and changes in dietary habits based on the results of a lipids profile blood test. The collective results indicated significantly improved cardiovascular and strength fitness scores, as well as reduced "bad" cholesterol and triglycerides. In addition, exercise adherence rates were well beyond most related studies, at approximately 70–76% for both aerobic and strength training. The Anshel et al. (2010) study included a measure of mental well-being. The researchers found significant gains in selected dimensions of mental health among participants.

Two case studies were conducted with a sedentary, obese, middle-aged male (Anshel, 2008) and a middle-aged male with strong religious convictions whose core values included faith (Anshel, 2010). In both case studies, the participants were asked to indicate three unhealthy habits from a list of 20 undesirable habits, including lack of exercise and poor nutrition. Then they listed the reasons for engaging in each negative habit, which formed the habit's "benefits", followed by the "costs" and "long-term consequences". It was important that the participant acknowledge that each of these behavior patterns was, in fact, unhealthy and undesirable; otherwise, he would find no reason to acknowledge their costs and seek to replace them with healthy routines. If lack of exercise was perceived as desirable, for instance, there would be no perceived need to replace this unhealthy habit with a more active lifestyle.

Participants were then asked to identify up to five core values that reflect their most important (core) beliefs about what really matters to them in living a high and happy quality of life. The second client (Anshel, 2010), who was a person of deep religious convictions, placed faith at the top of his list of values. The next step, particularly important, asked clients to identify an inconsistency, or disconnect, between the negative habits and values they had identified. The person of faith (Anshel, 2010) indicated that his obesity and unhealthy lifestyle were inconsistent with his value of faith, given the importance of maintaining healthy habits in Scripture. Other disconnects were found between values of character, health, and family as inconsistent with the unhealthy habits of lack of exercise, poor diet and nutrition, and low energy toward family and job. Both clients detected at least one disconnect between their values and behavior patterns.

The clients were then asked: "Given the costs and consequences of each unhealthy habit you found, is the disconnect acceptable?" Participants in both case studies acknowledged a disconnect between at least one of their values and a behavior pattern they deemed *undesirable* or *unhealthy*. They also indicated a strong desire to change the status quo by replacing their unhealthy habit with a more desirable one.

The clients were asked to what extent they were committed to work on and follow an action plan to remove the disconnect and to replace at least one of their unhealthy habits using a scale of 1 (*not at all committed*) to 10 (*extremely committed*); they both indicated "10" (i.e., extremely committed). An action plan was then constructed by the program's performance coach, who worked with a fitness coach and a registered dietician to follow through on changing the participant's exercise and dietary habits, respectively.

Results of both case studies demonstrated marked changes in fitness scores for upper and lower body strength, submax VO_2 exercise testing on a treadmill, and percent body fat (all *ps* $< .05$). The clients also reported changes in their diet based on adhering to the dietician's individualized program.

A poststudy debriefing indicated the clients' failure to acknowledge their self-destructive lifestyle; misalignment with their deepest values; the lack of energy from their current (unhealthy) lifestyle; and the need to be aware of their family's needs and others "who matter" such as work colleagues, their religious leaders, and friends in making significant changes in replacing their unhealthy habits. While the results of these case studies do not provide conclusive evidence of the model's efficacy, the participants did provide narratives, reported in the study, that reflected their strong commitment to health behavior change based on acknowledging their self-described "failure" to maintain healthier habits that are consistent with their values. Client attempts at generating and following an action plan that served to realign their habits with their most important values served as a strong motivator toward changing their daily habits, they reported.

Efficacy of the DVM was examined in an earlier (group) study by Anshel and Kang (2008). The researchers examined the model's efficacy in changing the unhealthy habits of 57 male and female police officers using an action research method. Action research is a reputable research method when situational conditions do not lend themselves to multiple group experimental designs, such as frequent interactions among study participants or the required use of programs or treatments that are publically advertised throughout the immediate environment, such as educational settings or, in this case, law enforcement. Action research consists of developing and implementing a plan of action without a control group. A control group which may not always be available nor appropriate to observe the effects of carrying out an action plan and to plan subsequent activities until predetermined goals are met (Mills, 2003).

The Anshel and Kang (2008) study began with a two-hour seminar that started the intervention covered in each stage of the DVM. The officers indicated their lifestyles were generally sedentary; they were unfit (i.e., they were not exercising nor engaging in regular vigorous physical activity), overweight, ate "fast food" at least once per day, suffered from poor sleep and chronic stress, and often experienced low physical energy. The officer's engaged in a 10-week action plan that consisted of fitness and nutrition coaching, in addition to meeting their performance coach—the seminar leader—on at least one occasion for an hour to review the overall action plan and to insert new routines that would improve adherence to exercise and dietary changes. They were given the option to meet individually for a second hour as a follow up, and 60% of the group opted for the second meeting. The results of the study indicated significantly improved scores ($ps < .01$) on submax VO_2 (cardio) and strength (upper and lower limb) fitness tests, lipids profile scores consisting of "good" and "bad" cholesterol levels, and reduced percent body fat.

To ensure that outcomes are a function of the treatment, action research includes several forms of validation including evaluative, outcome, and process validity. Each of these was evident in the Anshel and Kang (2008) study and in more recent similar studies conducted on a university campus (Anshel, Brinthaupt, & Kang, 2010; Anshel, Kang, & Brinthaupt, 2010). *Evaluative validity*, which addresses the objectivity of the quantitative nature of the data, is associated with significant improvements in fitness. *Outcome validity* is obtained from changes in specific behaviors that lead to successful outcomes under study and is applicable to future research (e.g., significant improvement from pretest to post-test). *Process validity* reflects correct execution of the intervention.

Taken together, it is apparent that earlier fitness intervention research attempts have been replete with limitations-such as imposing exercise locations, programs, schedules, and coaches-fail to develop social support coach-client relationships, and do not address lifestyle changes that integrate exercise with other healthy behavioral patterns such as nutrition, sleep, and stress management. Perhaps even more important in recognizing the limitations of past empirical attempts to change health behavior has been the absence of client values. The client's recognition of living a life filled with unhealthy habits that is *disconnected* from his or her values has been an enlightening, even life-changing observation.

Limitations of the DVM and Future Directions

While the results of previous studies and the reviewed conceptual frameworks lend credence to validating the DVM, further research that tests the model under various conditions, circumstances, and with different sample characteristics is warranted. Traditionally, research and practice of health behavior change have been concerned primarily with the psychological and behavioral factors that influence behavior. The role of noncredentialed consultants, such as fitness coaches and dieticians, are relatively rare in the related applied literature. The DVM provides an opportunity for individuals who are licensed (e.g., therapists, psychologists, social workers) and unlicensed (e.g., coaches, medical practitioners, consultants) in mental health to play a significant role in health behavior change. Examples include promoting physical activity; improving nutrition; promoting proper sleep patterns; overcoming injury or pain through effective rehabilitation techniques; and being able to manage stress, anxiety, and other undesirable emotions and feelings.

In addition, if mental health professionals have completed their degree program in a sport science, exercise science, kinesiology, or physical education program, they may have taken a course in exercise physiology or fitness. This background would be advantageous in developing an action plan for exercise clients and provide an additional source of social support, including prescribing an exercise routine and even exercising with the client. Experts in various areas of the action plan can be solicited and included in this phase of the model.

Researchers and practitioners concerned with health behavior change have suggested several avenues of future research. For instance, with respect to helping others develop an exercise habit, Baranowski et al. (1998) suggest that future research should focus on a better understanding of the *predictors* of physical activity and toward interventions that have demonstrated effectiveness in these predictors. Nicassio, Meyerowitz, and Kerns (2004) suggest that future studies include "specific methodologies for selecting intervention approaches in individual clinical cases" and acknowledge "the mechanisms of action through which interventions achieve their effects" (p. 135). One of these mechanisms might be the timespan between behavior and experiencing the payoffs from that behavior. In their study linking values and exercise behavior, for example, Segar et al. (2011) suggest that "because immediate payoffs motivate behavior better than distant goals, a more effective 'hook' for promoting sustainable participation might be to rebrand exercise as a primary way individuals can enhance the quality of their daily lives" (p. 94).

A key word in testing the DVM's efficacy is "mechanisms," that is, determining and understanding the specific reasons for the DVM's effectiveness in changing health behavior. Is it that people maintain their unhealthy habits without giving it a second thought and automatically self-destruct because these habits have been carried out in the virtual absence of conscious thought? Perhaps the DVM assists individuals to pay attention to their actions; to recognize that we pay a heavy price—called long-term consequences in the model—for these undesirable behaviors; and that our actions run counter to our deepest values, such as family, faith, health, character, and many others. Thinking through the long-term consequences of our actions is uncommon, primarily because we are a culture that rewards and recognizes immediate, rather than delayed, gratification.

The DVM embraces the need to examine the antecedents and clinical issues that affect the need to make healthy lifestyle changes, particularly in relation to promoting an exercise habit. This is one strategic approach to address possible ways to change behavior and prevent what is becoming a dangerous health crisis. New, creative approaches to changing health behavior are needed with a particular focus on examining the DVM's efficacy on initiating and adhering to regular exercise. A sedentary lifestyle is potentially fatal. As Glasgow et al. (2004) have concluded about future study of health behavior change, "If we are serious about evidence-based behavioral medicine and about closing the gap between research findings and application of these findings in applied settings, we cannot continue 'business as usual'" (p. 11).

References

Anshel, M.H. (2008). The Disconnected Values Model: Intervention strategies for health behavior change. *Journal of Clinical Sport Psychology*, *2*, 357–380.

Anshel, M.H. (2010). The Disconnected Values (Intervention) Model for promoting healthy habits in religious institutions. *Journal of Religion and Health*, *49*, 32–49.

Anshel, M.H., & Kang, M. (2007). An outcome-based action study on changes in fitness, blood lipids, and exercise adherence based on the Disconnected Values Model. *Behavioral Medicine*, *33*, 85–98.

Anshel, M.H., & Kang, M. (2008). Effectiveness of motivational interviewing on changes in fitness, blood lipids, and exercise adherence among police officers. *Journal of Correctional Health Care*, *14*, 48–62.

Anshel, M.H., Brinthaupt, T.M., & Kang, M. (2010). The Disconnected Values Model improves mental well-being and fitness in an employee wellness program. *Behavioral Medicine, 36*, 113–122.

Anshel, M. H., Kang, M., & Brinthaupt, T. M. (2010). Promoting health behavior change with the Disconnected Values Model: An action study. *International Journal of Sport and Exercise Psychology, 8*, 413–433.

Baranowski, T., Anderson, C., & Carmack, C. (1998). Mediating variable framework in physical activity interventions. How are we doing? How might we do better? *American Journal of Preventive Medicine, 15*, 266–297.

Festinger, L. (1957). *A theory of cognitive dissonance*. Stanford, CA: Stanford University Press.

Glasgow, R.E., Klesges, L.M., Dzewaltowski, D.A., Bull, S.S., & Estabrooks, P. (2004). The future of health behavior change research: What is needed to improve translation of research into health promotion practice. *Annals of Behavioral Medicine, 27*, 3–12.

Gollwitzer, P. M. (1999). Implementation intentions: Strong effects of simple plans. *American Psychologist, 54*, 493–503.

Lox, C.L., Martin Ginis, K.A., & Petruzzello, S.J. (2014). *The psychology of exercise: Integrating theory and practice* (4th ed.). Scottsdale, AZ: Holcomb Hathaway.

Nicassio, P. M., Meyerowitz, B.E., & Kerns, R.D. (2004). The future of health psychology interventions. *Health Psychology, 23*, 132–137.

Ossman, W.A., Wilson, K.G., Storaasli, R.D., & McNeill, J.W. (2006). A preliminary investigation of the use of Acceptance and Commitment Therapy in group treatment for social phobia. *International Journal of Psychology and Psychological Therapy, 6*, 397– 416.

Resnicow, K., Dilorio, C., Soet, J.E., Borrelli, B., Hecht, J., & Ernst, D. (2002). Motivational interviewing in health promotion: It sounds like something is changing. *Health Psychology, 21*, 444–451.

Resnicow, K., Jackson, A., Wang, T., Dudley, W., & Baranowski, T. (2001). A motivational interviewing intervention to increase fruit and vegetable intake through black churches: Results of the Eat for Life trial. *Journal of Cancer Education, 91*, 1686–1693.

Rollnick, S., Mason, P., & Butler, C. (1999). *Health behavior change: A guide for practitioners*. London: Churchill Livingstone.

Segar, M.L., Eccles, J.S., & Richardson, C.R. (2011). Rebranding exercise: closing the gap between values and behavior. *International Journal of Behavioral Nutrition and Physical Activity, 8*, 94–108.

PART III

Describing the Disconnected Values Model

6

NEGATIVE HABITS

Changing our habits, especially behaviors that we have ritualized over many years, is very challenging because the routines we embrace regularly, such as lack of regular exercise, poor nutrition, and bad dietary habits (e.g., having a bowl of ice cream before bedtime; replacing a proper meal with eating sweets) are firmly entrenched in our lifestyle. Unhealthy habits, however, may not be consistent with our values.

The model begins with this chapter to acknowledge our negative/unhealthy habits. The purpose of listing these habits is to help clients clearly identify their actions that might be called "self-destructive" if, in fact, the clients continue to act in ways that they know are contrary to their health and well-being. The identification process brings the client from behaving automatically and subconsciously to becoming self-aware of the unhealthy actions that, as shown later, have serious consequences.

One more reason to help clients identify their unhealthy habits is that many people are in denial about any habit that might be considered unhealthy or negative. They have engaged in unhealthy habits throughout their lifetime. It is understandably difficult for some individuals to acknowledge their lifestyle choices as not normal. Instead, many persons are protective of their lifestyle choices and ignore or discount the medical literature for making lifestyle changes (e.g., "My whole family is overweight; that's who we are" or "I've always been that way"). Having clients identify negative/unhealthy habits allows them to prioritize the unhealthy routines they want to change without appearing defensive or self-righteous.

Identifying Negative Habits

The DVM begins by helping the client acknowledge and identify habits—either specific routines or "regular" behavior patterns—that can be categorized as undesirable, unhealthy, or negative. These undesirable habits can be actions (e.g., lack of physical activity), thoughts (e.g., negative thinking, pessimism, criticism), or emotions (e.g., anger, negative mood) that occur "regularly," ranging from several times a day to every few days—long enough to have a deleterious effect on the person's health or well-being. It is assumed that these regularly experienced undesirable habits are under the person's control and, therefore, are susceptible to change. Despite our ability to prevent or stop these negative habits, we maintain them. Examples include impatience, daily sedentary behavior (i.e., lack of physical activity), poor nutrition, lack of hydration, excessive use of pharmaceutical agents, anger, and poor communication.

The following question should be asked when addressing an audience, a group DVM session, or an individual client: "Why do most of us do things every day that we know is bad (i.e., unhealthy, unpleasant, self-destructive) for us?" Researchers and theorists have attempted to understand this confusing tendency.

The primary reason most of us engage in negative habits is because we recognize the "benefits" of unhealthy habits and that these benefits outweigh the short-term costs and long-term consequences of maintaining the unhealthy habit (Hall & Fong, 2007). Hall and Fong claim, in their *temporal self-regulation theory*, that human behavior is driven by our need to meet immediate, not delayed, gratification (contingencies). An example would be the tendency of many people to avoid developing a daily exercise routine due to, they often contend, a lack of time to exercise. Researchers have found that "lack of time" is the highest ranked reason people claim they do not exercise regularly. As we will see later, the "perceived excuse" or "exercise barrier" of "no time" is just that—a perception. Good time management skills will always allow time for engaging in exercise and other forms of physical activity. In addition, individuals who do not regularly exercise often fail to understand that short-term "costs," that is, the time needed to exercise (or eat healthy or any other healthy habit), is the investment we make in experiencing the long-term benefits of regular exercise, such as improved energy, reduce risk of cardiovascular disease, and weight control.

Establishing an exercise habit is particularly challenging because it is often accompanied by negative feelings and attitudes that may have been based on earlier unpleasant experiences. For instance, with respect to developing an exercise habit, a previous physical education teacher may have used exercise as a form of discipline, or an athlete may feel burnout from too much physical training. Excessive or intense exercise may have contributed to a serious injury. To obtain desirable goals from exercise requires effort and even a degree of physical discomfort. Experiencing physical muscular fatigue, increasing heart rate, and overcoming poor fitness are very challenging for many (unfit) individuals. For some people, exercise can be financially costly if purchasing special clothing, particularly proper footwear, or exercising outdoors in the heat or cold. Memberships in fitness clubs or other facilities that promote various forms of physical activity (e.g., recreation centers, Boys and Girls Clubs) create further challenges to increasing an active lifestyle and reaching exercise goals. Mental health professionals, dieticians, and exercise coaches need interventions, such as the Disconnected Values Model, to overcome these barriers and improve the frequency and intensity of exercise participation and long-term adherence to exercise programs. The willingness to experience long-term benefits (e.g., good heart health) for short-term sacrifices (e.g., engaging in aerobic and resistance forms of training) is called *delayed gratification.*

Another example of delayed gratification concerns food intake. People who prefer a "fast food" meal, particularly if consumed daily, over a meal that is more nutritious, often more expensive, and takes longer to prepare are eating expediently to satisfy short-term needs. While the occasional "fast food" meal is relatively harmless in terms of poor nutrition, weight gain, increased "bad" cholesterol, and other undesirable outcomes, it is important to maintain a lifestyle in which food intake is based on delayed, not always immediate, gratification. Thus, one challenge to providing health care consulting is to help others understand the need to support and invest in *long-term benefits* of a healthy habit, rather than to focus on the false, short-term benefits.

Hall and Fong contend that unhealthy or undesirable (negative) habits do not exist without benefits. Negative habits, then, are initiated and maintained under two conditions: (a) the habit's benefits outweigh its costs, and (b) benefits are experienced in the short term, while costs and consequences are likely to be experienced in the distant future or long term. Cultures who prioritize the benefits of immediate gratification as opposed to delayed gratification nurture the decision to engage in meeting short-term, often unhealthy, needs.

Sample Negative Habits

It is often beneficial when applying the DVM that coaches and health counselors provide a list of items, or options, from which clients can select in determining their responses to questions that reveal deep-seated personal issues. Therefore, the DVM program provides a list of negative habits that may stimulate the recall of other habits that clients might otherwise not remember.

Coaches and therapists can obtain this information in different ways. Here are a few options.

(1) Have the client circle a maximal number—let's say three or four—of habits that interfere with optimal performance in no particular order of importance or seriousness.
(2) The client can rank the habits or insert one or more new unhealthy habits that are not listed.
(3) Set up the list in Likert-scale format in which each item (negative habit) is followed by numbers ranging from 1 (of minor importance/has little effect on health or mental well-being) to 5 (of great important/has a serious effect on health or mental well-being). For example:

1	2	3	4	5
Not Important	Somewhat	Moderate	Very Important	Extremely Important

TABLE 6.1 List of Frequent Negative Habits that Compromise Health, Mental Well-Being, or Effective Performance

1. Poor team player (usually self-focused, does not assist others, interested in own goals only)
2. Does not communicate well with supervisor and/or colleagues
3. Does not exercise or remain physically active
4. Procrastinates; does not plan; poor time management (circle one or more on this line)
5. Late to meetings; generally not punctual
6. Uses tobacco products (e.g., smoking, chewing tobacco) knowing its harmful effects
7. Poor communication skills; keeps feelings to self
8. Easily becomes disturbed or upset
9. Rigid and inflexible; must get own way
10. Discourteous; rude
11. Consumes the time of colleagues; talkative
12. Does not learn new technology; relies on old (and slower) ways of doing things
13. Poor sleep habits/insufficient sleep
14. Short attention span; poor concentration skills
15. No work/life balance; does not maintain an active personal life
16. Poor nutrition and hydration (poor food choices; insufficient water intake)
17. Does not take notes and have a calendar; relies on memory to complete tasks
18. Lack of trust in others
19. Lack of self-discipline and follow-through
20. Negative and pessimistic thinker; often critical
21. Impatient, impulsive
22. Failure to connect work to deepest values and beliefs
23. Low self-control
24. Lack of needed assertiveness and self-direction
25. Other: ______________________________
26. Other: ______________________________

Two important points need to be made here. First, remember that this component of the DVM addresses the performing of the client's negative habits, not the outcomes of these habits. This section concerns people's self-destructive actions that impede optimal performance, not the performance barriers that result from maintaining these habits. Performance barriers are the second component of the model (discussed later).

The second point concerns how to respond to clients who fail to locate a negative habit. While unlikely, ask the clients to tell you what they *do*, *feel*, or *think* on a "regular basis" that they know is unhealthy or undesirable—at least over time—even if they have acted this way for as long as they can remember. Do they have a quick temper? Do they act differently under pressure or treat others disrespectfully? Are they impatient? While lack of exercise, poor nutrition, lack of proper hydration, and poor sleep are typical negative habits and often experienced by most people, other tendencies are not as common.

Examples include low motivation, being self-critical or highly critical of others, feeling depressed or anxious over time (i.e., chronic depression or anxiety), speaking disrespectfully about others (e.g., supervisor, colleagues, the business or company), or maintaining a habit that others find annoying—or worse. If a client is in denial and refuses to divulge a negative habit, which is unlikely, ask the question "What would others find annoying or upsetting about something you do, and what is the cost to you of their feelings?"

Reference

Hall, P.A., & Fong, G.T. (2007). Temporal self-regulation theory: A model for individual health behavior. *Health Psychology Review*, *1*, 6–52.

7

PERFORMANCE BARRIERS

The initiation and continuation of negative/unhealthy habits eventually wear down the body's processes and result in a deterioration of health. Over time and with repetition, *negative habits lead to performance barriers.* Performance barriers are operationally defined as a persistent thought, emotion, or behavior that creates obstacles to good health and high-quality performance (Anshel, 2008). Performance barriers can be actual (e.g., injury, pain, anger, lack of facilities) or perceived (e.g., time restraints, lack of energy, mental discomfort, worry). The DVM considers performance barriers to always be under the person's control. For instance, the emotional barrier of anxiety (i.e., worry) can be controlled by addressing the source(s) of feeling threatened or worried and developing adaptation strategies that overcome these chronic (long term; persistent) or acute maladaptive thoughts (short term; isolated).

Performance barriers in the DVM have a root cause—negative habits. These behavioral tendencies, or habits, are labeled "negative" because: (a) it is generally acknowledged that they have a deleterious effect on some aspect of the person's quality of life and (b) that continued expression of the negative habits is directly linked to problems and limitations in work performance. For example, lack of exercise (or other forms of physical activity), which is commonly viewed as an unhealthy "physical" habit, may lead to low energy, premature mental fatigue, and obesity, among other outcomes. Persistent anxiety, an unhealthy "emotional" habit, may lead to poor (slow, inaccurate) decision making. The negative physical habit of poor work/life balance results in poor relationships with family, friends, and work colleagues.

One function of the model is to help clients detect their negative habits and how these habits lead to undesirable performance—physically, mentally, and emotionally—in various aspects of their life, not only health. The primary goal at this stage is that after negative habits have been associated with limitations to physical performance, the process begins in self-examining the *reasons* for maintaining negative habits such as lack of exercise.

Middle-aged persons who are uncomfortable and self-conscious about exercising among younger, fitter, thinner individuals at a fitness facility should focus on their exercise regimen, while ignoring others in the room. A person who has time restraints can develop time management strategies (e.g., brisk walking during the lunch hour or going for a walk, climbing stairs every 90 minutes, arranging coverage for your lunch-time responsibilities, early arrival to the fitness center twice a week) and implement social support (e.g., exercising with friends or a family member, scheduling coverage of job responsibilities with colleagues, working with a fitness coach or other professional).

The primary objectives for health professionals at this stage are: (1) to identify negative habits, (2) to associate these habits with limitations to physical performance, and (3) to begin the process of self-examining the reasons of maintaining negative habits. For instance, lack of sleep is a negative/unhealthy habit. Insufficient sleep might lead to poor concentration or slowing of information processing, thereby compromising memory. In another example, smoking is a negative habit (for multiple reasons regarding health, energy, and performance quality), but it becomes a performance barrier when others (e.g., work colleagues, family members, friends) choose not to interact with the smoker or when a smoking addiction disturbs sleep, proper nutrition, concentration, and work performance and leads to ill health. Barriers impede the flow of energy, performance effectiveness, and quality of life.

One would think that it's easy to designate areas of one's life that are accompanied by struggle and anguish. Designating barriers should be a relatively easy task, but that is not always the case. The challenge to coaches and health professionals in designating performance barriers is the client's *denial, defensiveness, and lack of self-awareness* that barriers even exist or that they are of minimal importance that do not warrant time and attention in this program. Denial, defensiveness, and lack of self-awareness work interchangeably to *impede* discovering "the truth" about the level of importance of events and issues (i.e., barriers to experiencing happiness, life satisfaction, and optimal performance) that need work and change.

Table 7.1 lists possible barriers that compromise good health, improved quality of life, and/or performance. Have clients designate up to five barriers, preferably the most important ones that might rate "9" or "10" on a 10-point scale. The ability to designate barriers is the starting point toward expanding our mental, emotional, and spiritual capacity to think and meet our need to change and get better.

Designating performance barriers, which follows designating negative habits in the model, is important because: (1) these barriers provide insights into the selection and application of rituals that address the barriers; (2) labeling the barriers

TABLE 7.1 Barriers that Compromise Good Health, Quality of Life, and High Quality Performance. *Circle up to five barriers that describe your life (unranked).*

1. Lack of assertiveness and self-direction
2. Poor team player (thinks "me" not "we")
3. Constant conflict with boss or coworker
4. Poor fitness
5. Poor organization and time management
6. Low motivation and passion at work
7. Fear and insecurity on the job
8. Poor communication skills
9. Low stress tolerance; easily stressed or upset
10. Rigid and inflexible
11. Poor sleep habits (e.g., late bedtime hour, eating or exercise before sleep)
12. Low energy
13. Physical fatigue
14. Mental fatigue
15. Poor work/life balance (lack of personal life)
16. Poor nutrition and hydration
17. Lack of trust in others
18. Lack of discipline and follow through
19. Lack of empathy and compassion
20. Lack of integrity and good character
21. Negative and pessimistic thinker
22. Impatience, frustration, and anger
23. Failure to connect work to deepest values and beliefs
24. Poor relationships in personal life
25. Low self-control over own actions
26. Short attention span
27. Poor concentration
28. High anxiety
29. Pessimistic/negative thinker (anticipates failure or not meeting goals)
30. Lack of passion
31. Moody/irritable/frequent ups and downs
32. Forgetful
33. Other (your selection): ______________________________

____

motivates clients to examine the costs and consequences of their negative habits; and (3) designating performance barriers allow coaches and mental health professionals the opportunity to develop effective action plans for clients and to measure desirable changes, including the elimination of these barriers. Thus, performance barriers serve a motivational function in encouraging clients to replace at least some of their undesirable habits with "positive" and healthier rituals. After performance barriers have been designated, clients are asked to examine the reasons they maintain unhealthy habits by looking at the benefits, costs, and consequences of their actions.

Reference

Anshel, M.H. (2008). The Disconnected Values Model: Intervention strategies for health behavior change. *Journal of Clinical Sport Psychology*, *2*, 357–380.

8

PERCEIVED BENEFITS, COSTS, AND CONSEQUENCES

This is a crucial component of the model in the attempt to change unhealthy habits. In this segment of the model, we return to the question about why people tend to do things that they know are bad (i.e., unhealthy, negative) for them—sometimes daily. Why are we sometimes so self-destructive in our daily habits? We know, for instance, that a sedentary lifestyle, eating certain foods in excess, and drinking alcohol or soft drinks excessively are all very unhealthy and lead to undesirable consequences. And, yet, we continue to drink or eat these same substances and accept the undesirable consequences, even death. We consciously behave in ways one might call "irresponsible" and against our own best interests. Why? Researchers have studied the causes of self-destructive behaviors. There are *perceived* benefits to each of our unhealthy habits, such as lack of exercise or other forms of physical activity, or else the unhealthy habit would not continue.

It is important to recognize the term "perceived" in this context because a person who repeatedly and habitually engages in unhealthy, self-destructive behavior patterns is able to justify his or her actions, either rationally (e.g., to quickly satisfy hunger, not enough time to exercise) or irrationally (e.g., "I am obese, but my doctor tells me I am healthy and I'm just fine"). Perception, then, is in the eye of the beholder and reflects the individual's sense of reality. Thus, one's perception does not necessarily represent reality, in this case, medical test data or the opinion of the person's medical practitioner that the patient hears (versus other medical advice the patient ignores or discounts).

As discussed earlier, the "benefits" of not exercising, for example, include more time to do other things and not experiencing the discomfort of training, the exertion, and the expenses related to purchasing fitness club memberships and exercise clothing. It is crucial in the DVM that the client list—verbally or in writing—the so-called benefits, or advantages, to maintaining a particular habit that may be labeled "negative" or not in the person's best interests. These benefits help explain the person's persistence in continuing to retain the habit on a regular basis—daily, weekly, monthly. If the person perceives no benefits to the unhealthy habit, then the habit should become meaningless and irrelevant. A listing of one or more benefits balances the next phase of this process—listing the habit's short-term costs and long-term consequences.

Costs and Long-Term Consequences of Negative (Unhealthy) Habits

The corporate community is familiar with the concept of a cost-benefit tradeoff, that is, the process by which decisions are made based on listing the benefits—the upside—and the costs—the downside. At this stage, the client is asked to recognize the downside, or sacrifices, that are made in maintaining the negative/unhealthy habits. In our exercise example, the benefits of not exercising or engaging in other forms of regular physical activity are balanced out by short-term *costs* and long-term *consequences*.

A few costs of a sedentary lifestyle include poor cardiovascular and strength fitness, weight gain, higher stress and anxiety, reduced physical energy, lower mental (cognitive) functioning, and less satisfactory sleep. The long-term "consequences" of not exercising include poorer physical and mental health; depression; a higher probability of diseases such as diabetes, certain cancers, and cardiovascular disease; reduced quality of life; and a shorter lifespan (Long & van Stavel, 1995; Stathopoulou, Powers, Berry, Smits, & Otto, 2006). Again, as is the case with the "benefits" list, listing the costs and consequences is optimally effective if it comes from the client and is not a coach-generated list.

The client is then asked a very important question that should have high self-motivation value: *"Despite the so-called benefits of this negative habit, are the short-term costs and long-term consequences of this negative habit acceptable to you? Are you prepared to live with these costs and consequences?"*

If the client concludes that the costs of a particular negative, unhealthy habit are indeed acceptable, then the negative habit (e.g., not exercising, maintaining a sedentary lifestyle, temperamental, chronic anxiety, poor nutrition) will likely continue. If, however, the costs or consequences are *greater* than the benefits of maintaining the unhealthy habit, *and* the person concludes that these costs are *unacceptable*, then a change in behavior is far more likely.

The model posits that the process of behavior change is not yet complete, however. Missing is the *ignition point* that links the costs of inactivity to the person's deepest values and beliefs—the client's values—and that is explained in the next chapter. Table 8.1 provides examples of perceived benefits, costs, and long-term consequences of selected negative habits. Coaches may want to have clients fill in their own response set (leave a set of blank boxes).

TABLE 8.1 Benefits, Costs, and Long-Term Consequences of Negative Habits

	Current Habit	*Benefits*	*Costs*	*Long-Term Consequences*
1	Negative attitude, pessimistic, anticipation of failure	Less disappointment, less risk of failure, less vulnerability, less effort, attempt to escape blame, takes no responsibility for task outcome	Reduced positive energy, low motivation, higher stress, less effective immediate performance	Poor health and long-term performance, reduced life satisfaction and happiness, lower group cohesion
2	Poor work/life balance	Accomplish more at work, less emotional risk, avoid responsibilities outside of work, ignore or limited time with family	Lack of time for intimate connection with friends and family, poor work efficiency	Unfulfilling relationships, tendency to impatience and anger, burnout, regret, guilt, loss of passion
3	Anger and impatience	Prompts action, discharges tension	Antagonizes colleagues, begets more anger	Demotivating, antagonizing to others, undermines close relationships, increases health risks
4	Disengagement from tasks, relationships, and obligations	Reduces anxiety, avoids taking responsibility for failure, lower perceived failure, less stress	Reduces passion for work and personal relationships, poor connection to others, undermines performance	Shallow life, lack of meaning, low achievement, reduced performance quality
5	Poor recovery from stress	Accomplish more in the short-term, feeling productive, fulfills need for work and task completion	Fatigue, reduced passion and performance, higher health risks	Poor health, higher rate of burnout, less energy, undermines relationships, diminishes performance
6	Poor sleep	More tasks to be productive, fulfills need to achieve, put more hours into job	Lack of concentration, mental and physical fatigue by midday, reduced immune system effectiveness	Superficial connection to others, less capacity for focusing on primary goal(s), lower quality of work, poor concentration, sickness

7	Poor diet (high fat, high sugar)	Immediate gratification, convenience, low cost, good tasting food, fast service	High cholesterol, increased weight, less sustained energy, increases likelihood for various diseases	Increased risk of obesity, heart disease, strokes, cancer, diabetes, purchasing expensive medicines, and early death
8	Frustration, impatience, anger, defensiveness toward others	Keeps people at a safe distance, avoids responsibility, maintains control	Alienates coworkers, undermines teamwork, negative mood.	Isolation, rigidity, poor relationships, failure to grow and improve quality of work, leads to burnout
9	Excessive alcohol and drug abuse	Immediate pleasure, reduced tension and anxiety, easier to socialize with others	Impaired concentration, erratic work performance, dangerous for driving and breaking the law, mood swings, inappropriate behavior	Higher health risks, undermines relationships, self-esteem and performance
10	No exercise/sedentary lifestyle	More time for work and other obligations, less effort and experiencing exertion and physical fatigue, not spending money on exercise clothing and fitness club memberships	Less energy, strength, general well-being; no recovery from mental activities, reduced concentration, more susceptibility to sickness	Undermines health, lowers concentration and energy, increases chances of diseases and early death

It is crucial, in this stage, that most of the answers about identifying the "benefits," "costs," and "consequences" of each negative habit (or as many habits as the client and coach wish to address) come from the client and not, if at all possible, from the coach/therapist. Client-generated responses make this task far more meaningful and personal for the client than if a coach or therapist supplied these responses. The possible exception to a client-centered procedure is when a coach needs to prompt clients who are not able or who are hesitant to generate their own responses.

For example, client Dave agreed that his tendency to be a perfectionist and to spend between 70–80 hours a week at his job in the financial industry was fine with him because "that's who I am." It would be meaningless to coerce Dave to acknowledge that there are costs and consequences to a self-imposed 80-hour work week when the client sees and prioritizes the benefits of his work schedule. Therefore, Dave's work schedule was not necessarily a negative habit—through his eyes. What *was* a negative habit was not his work habit but rather his failure to engage with his two sons, who were now in their thirties and all grown up without establishing a relationship with their father. That aspect of a self-imposed heavy work schedule—losing touch with his sons and not having a role in their upbringing—was clearly meaningful to Dave and was not acceptable to him. He wanted to recapture what he missed as they grew and developed as young men. Now that they were already grown (but neither had yet married), he wanted to know them and develop the relationship he never had with each son. It was this aspect of his life that created the foundation of a disconnect between his values and his "negative" habit of overworking.

The power of this stage cannot be overstated. It is essential that clients first be able to identify habits they consider unhealthy, undesirable, and warranting change—either a reduction or the elimination of the unhealthy habit. Then it is essential that they work with the coach/therapist to review the "benefits" of this habit so they understand the reasons the habit is maintained. Unless benefits of an unhealthy habit are reviewed, it will be difficult to contrast them with the other side of this ledger—the costs and long-term consequences of the undesirable habit. Identification of benefits brings the negative habit into reality. The client says, "Oh, yes, now I know the reasons for overeating . . ." or "I remember why I have become such a perfectionist and so critical of others. . . . It's because my extremely high expectations of others reflects how I was treated growing up and the gratification I felt from achieving more and more."

Clients must be informed that "excessive, self-serving behavior" carries risks to one's health and happiness. "Sure, as the business owner you can bully and make very high and repressive demands on your employees, but here's the cost: you'll lose their loyalty, their self-motivation to help the company, and their feelings to be part of a team in which all employees pull together to improve performance and profits. Is that ok with you?" Clients must understand that making poor choices carries risks to one's health, happiness, and life satisfaction. This information is then carried over to the next stage, identifying one's core values.

References

Long, B. C., & van Stavel, R. (1995). Effects of exercise training on anxiety: A meta-analysis. *Journal of Applied Sport Psychology*, 7, 167–189.

Stathopoulou, G., Powers, M.B., Berry, A.C., Smits, J.A., & Otto, M.W. (2006). Exercise interventions for mental health: A Quantitative and qualitative review. *Clinical Psychology: Science and Practice*, *13*,179–193.

9

VALUES

All of us have areas of our lives that we hold sacrosanct, that is, thoughts, emotions, and actions—core beliefs—that give us purpose and meaning. To Rokeach (1973), these core beliefs that guide and motivate behavior and provide standards against which we judge ourselves are called values (Rokeach, 1973). For example, as Rokeach contends, a person who considers safety and freedom to be important values will tend to act in ways that reduce risk to one's well-being. In addition, most people develop daily rituals that help ensure that their values, such as safety and freedom, are maintained. To Hogan and Mookherjee (1981), "the likely effects of values on human behavior, beliefs, and attitudes are indisputable" (p. 29).

While most of us possess values that are intended to guide behavior, the relationship between values and behaviors that support these values are not always consistent. There may be a misalignment between one's values and behavior patterns. For instance, Segar, Eccles, and Richardson (2011) found that the relationship between the goals and core values of 226 middle-aged female exercisers, ranging in age from 40–60 years, was relatively low. That is, there was a significant discrepancy between the exercisers' goals and values. They concluded that exercise goals related to health and healthy aging were associated *less* with exercise than those related to enhancing daily quality of life, despite being equally valued. This finding provides further evidence for developing an exercise intervention that promotes a consistency between our values and our behavior patterns, in this case health and exercise, respectively.

While there is a paucity of research on the influence of values on exercise behavior, values tend to predict behavior (Hogan & Mookherjee, 1981), including regularly engaging in various forms of physical activity, such as exercise

(Brown & Crace, 1996). For example, it is likely that individuals who consider health an important value are more likely to maintain habits that promote good health than individuals who do not consider health among their most important values. Too often, however, the consistency between values (e.g., health) and behavior (e.g., unhealthy habits) is not found. Instead, persons who consider health as a relevant value often maintain an unhealthy lifestyle (e.g., poor nutrition, sedentary lifestyle, poor sleep, high stress). Tobacco users may acknowledge that tobacco use is unhealthy and they "should quit," or overweight individuals admit they need to lose weight and eat "healthier" yet maintain their old habit of overeating. These individuals demonstrate an inconsistency, misalignment, or disconnect between their values and their behavior patterns. In the DVM, it is imperative for the therapist/coach to obtain from clients their deepest values in order to determine evidence of a disconnect between the client's values and unhealthy habits.

The Importance of Values in Exercise Interventions

As indicated earlier, values are core beliefs that guide behavior, provide impetus for motivating behavior, and provide standards against which we assess behavior (Rokeach, 1973). Values are highly relevant to establishing a person's individuality and help our understanding of behavior. For example, as Rokeach contends, a person who values health will tend to develop daily rituals and long-term habits that enhance health and general well-being. Hogan and Mookherjee (1981) describe values as "one of the most distinguishing characteristics motivating human beings; the likely effects of values on human behavior, beliefs, and attitudes are indisputable" (p. 29).

Values are more central determinants of behavior than are interests and attitudes, the latter of which are more situational and derived from a core set of values (Super, 1995). Thus, a plethora of interests and attitudes are derived from a relatively reduced number of values. In addition, interests, attitudes, and needs are transitory and, once satiated, may not influence behavior. Values, on the other hand, are almost always firmly entrenched and stable and therefore transcend situations and guide behavior over a long period of time.

If you were to give individuals a list of values—what they consider to be their beliefs about what is really important to them—and then ask them to rank these values, health, family, character, and faith would likely be common, having been influenced by the person's culture and geographic location. Perhaps integrity, happiness, honesty, knowledge, performance excellence, commitment, integrity, and concern for others would be other highly rated choices (Loehr & Schwartz, 2003). Thus, behavior change is more likely to be permanent when the client concludes that life satisfaction is linked to behaving in a way that is consistent with one's deepest values.

Coach and Therapist Actions

Health practitioners should conduct the following tasks:

(1) Provide your client with the list of values (listed below), that is, a list of core beliefs that he or she considers to be really important and that reflect how to live.

(2) Start with their identification of three to five of their most important values. Having clients rank these values is optional. Some therapists do not see the relevance in ranking, as long as the client views each value as important. Frequent values would be health, family, character, and faith. The person's culture, geographic location, and other personal characteristics will often influence this list of values, but there is not a "right" or "wrong" answer to this question; all values are equally important if this is the client's choice. Thus, behavior change is more likely to be permanent when the client concludes that happiness and general well-being are linked to behaving in a way that is consistent with one's deepest values.

Values Checklist: Check three to five of your most important values

Authenticity	❐	Happiness	❐
Balance	❐	Harmony	❐
Beauty	❐	Health	❐
Character	❐	Honesty	❐
Commitment	❐	Humility	❐
Compassion	❐	Humor	❐
Concern for others	❐	Integrity	❐
Creativity	❐	Kindness	❐
Empathy	❐	Knowledge	❐
Excellence	❐	Loyalty	❐
Fairness	❐	Perseverance	❐
Faith	❐	Respect for others	❐
Family	❐	Responsibility	❐
Freedom	❐	Security	❐
Friendship	❐	Serenity	❐
Generosity	❐	Service to others	❐
Genuineness	❐	Wealth	❐
Other ________	❐		

References

Brown, D., & Crace, R.K. (1996). Values in life role choices and outcomes: A conceptual model. *Career Development Quarterly*, *44*, 21–223.

Hogan, H.W., & Mookherjee, H.N. (1981). Values and selected antecedents. *Journal of Social Psychology*, *113*, 29–35.

Loehr, J., & Schwartz, T. (2003). *The power of full engagement: Managing energy, not time, is the key to high performance and personal renewal.* New York: Free Press.

Rokeach, M. (1973). *The nature of human values.* New York: Free Press.

Segar, M.L., Eccles, J.S., & Richardson, C.R. (2011). Rebranding exercise: closing the gap between values and behavior. *International Journal of Behavioral Nutrition and Physical Activity, 8*, pp. 94–108.

Super, D. E. (1995). Values: Their nature, assessment, and practical use. In D.E. Super & B. Sverko (Eds.), *Life's roles, values, and careers: International findings of the work importance study* (pp. 54–61). San Francisco: Jossey-Bass.

10

DISCONNECTS BETWEEN NEGATIVE HABITS AND CORE VALUES

The next phase of the DVM is the heart of changing health behavior, that is, helping clients detect a disconnect, or inconsistency, between their values and at least one of their negative (unhealthy) habits. This section includes very carefully worded statements; therefore, this part of the DVM includes specific suggested narrative.

The following questions might be asked by the attending therapist or coach: "Joan, let's review the most important values that you checked in the previous phase (*coach reviews each value along with an action that supports—is consistent with—that value*).

> *Sample Client Interaction*: "To what extent are your values consistent with your actions?" The coach now offers the client an example. "For example, you indicated that ____ is one of your most important values. I want you to think about and tell me about a certain action or behavior pattern that you do regularly—perhaps daily—that you know is not good for you and is inconsistent with this value."
>
> *A specific example*: One of your values is health. This means that you strongly believe in maintaining proper health and well-being; healthy habits are desirable and good for you. Can you tell me what you do regularly that is not consistent with this value? Do you have any unhealthy habits? And why do you maintain this habit that you recognize is unhealthy?"

At this point, the coach must be prepared to offer clients possible examples of their unhealthy habits if they do not generate their own. Perhaps the client leads a sedentary lifestyle and does not exercise or perform other forms of physical activity (e.g., bicycling, walking, playing sports, gardening) on a regular basis. You might say, "One of your deepest values is to maintain good health; however, you do not engage in regular physical activity, you lead a sedentary lifestyle, and you chew tobacco/smoke. Can you see how your stated value of 'health' is inconsistent with your actions of living a sedentary lifestyle? Can you detect a 'disconnect' between your beliefs about good health and at least one of your unhealthy behavioral patterns? What other specific disconnects between your values and behaviors can *you* find?"

At this point, assuming clients acknowledge at least one disconnect between any of their values and one or more unhealthy habits, the coach then goes to the next stage: to review the short-term costs and long-term consequences of the disconnect.

Acceptability of the Disconnect

The process of health behavior change in the DVM collapses unless clients can *detect and accept* a disconnect between at least one (or more) of their values and at least one unhealthy (or negative) habit or behavior pattern. For instance, clients must acknowledge that the negative habit of not engaging in exercise or some other form of vigorous physical activity is inconsistent with their deepest values and beliefs about the value of health—IF, that is, they listed health as one of their deepest values. The follow-up question must be to ascertain if this is acceptable.

> "There are many reasons that explain why you do not exercise or engage in other forms of physical activity on a regular basis. You may not enjoy it, you may not have time, or there may not be a location for exercise that appeals to you or existing physical activity locations seem too far away, cost too much to join, or do not have an environment or physical conditions that attract you. Can you tell me (or write down) your particular reason for not exercising? It's not a 'right' or 'wrong' question; just state whatever you think.
>
> There are, however, costs and consequences for remaining inactive and not including various forms of physical activity among your daily habits. Let's review, quickly, some of these costs and long-term consequences."

In Anshel and Kang's (2008) study of validating the DVM in law enforcement, the male and female police officers indicated their lifestyles were generally sedentary and they were unfit (i.e., they were not exercising nor engaging in regular vigorous physical activity), overweight, ate "fast food" at least once per day, suffered from poor sleep and chronic stress, and often experienced low physical energy. After the officers recognized the disconnects between the unhealthy lifestyles and their values of family, health, faith, and quality of work performance, the officer's engaged in a 10-week action plan. The plan consisted of fitness and nutrition coaching, in addition to meeting their performance coach—the seminar leader—on at least one occasion for an hour to review their overall action plan and to insert new routines that would improve adherence to exercise and dietary changes. The results of the study indicated significantly improved fitness scores for both cardio and strength (upper and lower limb) fitness tests, lipids profile (i.e., cholesterol) scores, and reduced percent body fat.

In a case study, Anshel (2008) asked an adult male of faith to acknowledge the misalignment between his values, in which faith was ranked first, and his unhealthy habits of overeating, lack of physical activity, poor sleep, and negative relationships with family members. He was a regular participant in religious services, in which his religious text often reflected the virtues of healthy living. His behaviors, however, were completely inconsistent with this spiritual life. In this case, with his permission, specific passages from Scripture, which were consistent with his affiliation, were identified and presented to him. He immediately understood that the disconnect between his values and actions were preventing him from living a more joyous and fulfilled life, while lacking the energy and temperament needed to demonstrate love for his family, to bring honor to his religious leader, and to be consistent with his spiritual beliefs and actions.

At this time, the coach reviews the short-term costs and long-term consequences obtained from the client's chart that was completed earlier. If health is not one of the client's deepest values, or the client fails to identify a disconnect between the value of health and an unhealthy habit, then *the coach must find a new value and a different behavior pattern in which the client is more likely to find the disconnect.* The bottom line is that there are consequences for certain behaviors that is generally recognized as undesirable/negative/unhealthy. The DVM's effectiveness rests on finding that (those) disconnect(s).

Clients who refuse or are unable to identify a disconnect might be in denial and, consequently, may need professional counseling or psychotherapy. Readers who are not credentialed to provide counseling services might need to have a list of properly trained individuals available to whom they can refer a client. Clients may need credentialed and professionally trained therapists to examine evidence of unhealthy habits, values, and disconnects or inconsistencies between them so they can help clients reduce their denial and defensiveness in relation to undesirable behavior patterns. Defensiveness, irrational thinking, insecurity, and low self-esteem are just a few plausible reasons for lacking the proper level of objectivity in examining and identifying self-destructive behaviors.

In the absence of the client's ability to identify disconnects, coaches must ask clients to give some thought to the concept of an inconsistency between their values and actions, even to discuss this issue further at a subsequent meeting. It is also important to recognize that completing the action plan, in the next phase of the DVM, will address these so-called unhealthy habits in which the client might find the disconnect inconsequential. The key outcome here is that unhealthy habits are reduced or stopped and replaced by healthier and more desirable alternatives.

Any identified disconnects, however, must be originated by clients, perhaps with an assist by the coach, if needed.

Let's review this important phase of the model using the value of health and the behavior pattern of no exercise and a sedentary lifestyle. The coach must ask the client this important question: "Is the disconnect between the value of health and the negative habit of lack of exercise and a person feels passionate about acceptable to you? Is it ok, especially after knowing the costs and long-term consequences of this negative habit?"

If the disconnect *is* acceptable—and for many individuals who feel that changing the negative habit is either undesirable or beyond their control—then no change in the unhealthy habit (i.e., exercise behavior) will likely continue to occur. It would be necessary, therefore, to identify another disconnect between the person's values and at least one other negative habit. Only when a particular disconnect is unacceptable to the individual is the client prepared to commit to behavior change and then engage in developing and carrying out an action plan.

For example, the therapist asks the client, "Given the disconnect between your negative habit of not engaging in regular exercise and the costs and long-term consequences of this disconnect, is this acceptable to you? Is this ok?" If the client acknowledges the costs and long-term consequences of the disconnect and concludes the disconnect *is acceptable*, the client's negative habits will not change. If the disconnect is *unacceptable*, however, then the client may be ready to engage in an *action plan* that replaces the negative habit with one or more positive, healthier routines.

It is important to remember that negative habits and values are often linked to the client's culture, gender, education level, and other demographic characteristics. Coaches/therapists need to use the negative habit and value(s) that the client identifies as important; the client must not be expected to fit a habit that the coach/therapist thinks is important. The process must be "client-friendly." Clients must render their full support of each stage of the model so they commit to the last segment—the action plan.

References

Anshel, M.H. (2010). The Disconnected Values (Intervention) Model for promoting healthy habits in religious institutions. *Journal of Religion and Health*, *49*, 32–49.

Anshel, M.H., & Kang, M. (2008). Effectiveness of motivational interviewing on changes in fitness, blood lipids, and exercise adherence among police officers. *Journal of Correctional Health Care*, *14*, 48–62.

11

DETERMINING AND CARRYING OUT AN ACTION PLAN

Developing a Self-Regulation Action Plan

In this final stage of the model (long-term adherence strategies to ritualize the new habit notwithstanding), the client is now ready, with the guidance of his/her coach or therapist, to develop an action plan. The action plan begins the process of eliminating inconsistencies between values and unhealthy habit(s). Researchers and therapists know that developing new habits, or routines, requires time—weeks or months—to make automatic. Issues that need to be addressed include the time, location, and other conditions for the new habit(s) to emerge and become consistent. The person's decision to initiate an exercise program, for instance, should result in a permanent change in one's daily routine to accompany the time, location, and resources needed to maintain this new habit. Coaches want to help clients overcome the disconnect between their sedentary lifestyle (i.e., lack of exercise) and their value of (maintaining good) health.

After obtaining the client's (and, perhaps their physician's) approval and commitment to start a new exercise program of exercise—or other type of physical activity—the coach/therapist and client jointly develop a detailed self-regulation action plan.

Developing an action plan consists of designating the *type of activity*, *scheduling the time, location, conditions*, and additional details about putting the client's commitment into action (e.g., to exercise regularly). Action plan specifics, written out in detail, include the type of physical activity (e.g., exercise, bicycling, sport participation) and the time, days of the week, and location for performing this/these activities daily and weekly. More detailed planning is needed for on-site activities such as types, repetitions, and distance or minutes of exercises; whether to hire a personal trainer; inclusion and scheduling of exercise testing to establish a baseline of fitness and other health indicators; and availability of social support (e.g., exercising with others, sharing transportation to an exercise venue, securing the location), and ensuring that personal and professional needs and obligations have been addressed. Specificity of timing and precision of behavior dramatically increases the probability of successfully carrying out a self-controlled action plan (Anshel, 2014). The self-regulation action plan serves the primary purpose of creating a more immediate payoff and providing clients with a sense of achievement and improvement, among other immediate payoffs that have higher motivation value than using more distant goals (Segar, Eccles, & Richardson, 2011).

The action plan consists primarily of *three factors* that ostensibly promotes the client's *long-term* commitment to initiating and maintaining a new habit. Using exercise as an example: (1) determine a specific time within a 24-hour period for exercise engagement; (2) develop a set of routines that support the exercise habit (e.g., selected thoughts and behaviors prior to, during, and following the exercise session; exercising with a friend and promoting other forms of social support; minimizing distractions that will interfere with exercise plans), and (3) link the new habit to the client's deepest values and beliefs about the desire to eliminate the existing inconsistency between his or her values and current negative (undesirable) habit. Following are sample rituals that promote behavior change in replacing unhealthy habits with more desirable rituals. In the following example, we identify the concept, first developed by Loehr and Schwartz (2003), of expanding our capacity to go beyond current levels and to advance to a new level of achievement.

Important Rituals to Expand Physical Capacity

Circle the new routine(s) you are prepared to begin and insert the starting date and time.

Nutrition and Hydration **Starting Date and Time** (write below next to ritual) Example: Starts 1–5–15 at noon

1. Eat three meals and two snacks daily.

   ____

2. Eat breakfast daily.

   ____

3. Never go longer than four hours without food.

   ____

4. Eat 40% grains, 40% fruits and vegetables, and 20% protein.

   ____

5. Eat no more than five handfuls of food per meal (portion control).

   ____

6. Snacks should be 100 to 150 calories; include fruit. Snacking is a healthy habit.

   ___

7. Eighty percent of food intake at any meal will consist of *need* foods and 20% from *want* foods.

   ___

8. Eat until you are satisfied, not full or "stuffed."

   ___

9. Drink water regularly throughout the day, preferably 64 oz. or more.

   ___

10. Alcohol, if consumed, should be with meals; consume two glasses/day maximum.

    ___

11. Keep caffeinated beverages to a minimum and do not consume within three hours of bedtime.

    ___

Exercise and Other Forms of Physical Activity

1. Every 30 to 45 minutes, perform small movements.

   ___

2. Every 90 to 120 minutes, perform major movements.

   ___

3. Go to bed early and wake up early.

   ___

4. Do some form of physical activity daily.

   ___

5. Do at least two strength training workouts per week.

   ___

6. Do at least two cardiovascular interval workouts per week.

   ___

7. To expand capacity, expend energy to the feeling of discomfort.

   ___

8. Breathe from the diaphragm to enhance energy recovery.

   ___

9. Exercise at moderate to high intensity to improve cardiovascular capacity and burn more calories.

   ___

10. Ideal exercise length is 30–60 minutes, 3–5 times per week.

 ____

11. MOVE: Avoid prolonged sitting. Walk around or do something physical at least every 90 minutes. Recent research shows that sitting six or more hours per day predicts a cardiovascular event (heart attack, stroke).

 ____

One of the more important outcomes of an action plan and the foundation of promoting good health is improved sleep. While many individuals are sleep deprived (for any one of numerous reasons), there are rituals that can be applied that will facilitate high quality sleep. At least some, if not most, of these can be an integral part of the client's action plan.

Presleep and Sleep Rituals

Please check the starting dates and times for as many of these presleep rituals you can incorporate into your nightly schedule.

1. Go to bed and wake up consistently at the same times.

 ____

2. Sleep is usually higher quality earlier at night; "early to bed, early to rise."

 ____

3. Get seven to eight hours of sleep each night. Highly fit individuals may require less.

 ____

4. Avoid full meals within two hours of bedtime.

 ____

5. Avoid caffeine and alcohol within two hours of bedtime (they are diuretics, which increase arousal and urinary output, disturbing sleep).

 ____

6. Avoid stress, if at all possible, at least for two hours before bedtime.

 ____

7. Be aware of sleep apnea (cessation of breathing during sleep, often reflected by excessive and loud snoring during sleep and feeling fatigue upon awakening); apnea predicts stroke and heart attack.

 ____

8. Do something relaxing that eliminates unpleasant feelings and unpleasant feelings and reduces arousal level, such as reading, going for a walk, or slow and deep breathing. Avoid using a computer or other electronic device near bedtime due to its arousal-inducing effects.

 ____

9. Avoid watching television in your bedroom. According to the National Sleep Foundation, television increases somatic arousal (i.e., feelings of excitation) through higher heart rate and adrenaline.

---

10. "Act as if . . .": Our actions dictate our physiology and are more important for influencing a person's emotions and mood than thoughts alone. If, for example, you jumped up and down while yelling "I'm miserable, I'm miserable," you'd likely laugh and feel positive. This is because the jumping action is more powerful than words or thoughts. Therefore, "act as if" you feel good and full of energy. When you walk through the door at work you are "on." No one needs to know you did not sleep well (no one cares, anyway). Act upbeat and professional. Keep up a positive frame of mind and *act as if* you are in a positive mood state. You WILL feel better as a result.

Time Management Action Plan Schedule Components

The last segment of the client DVM session consists of scheduling the action plan. Note that the final phase of the model goes beyond establishing the plan; it's called "action plan adherence," which will be discussed separately. This phase of the action plan is called "time management" because it consists of establishing a detailed set of routines over a 24-hour period that are repeated and become one or more long-term, perhaps permanent, rituals. Some clients will feel very uncomfortable with detailed plans of their new routines; it represents a very structured day to ensure that new rituals are carried out as planned. Some individuals prefer more flexibility and not to be too structured. Everyone is different in how to implement the plan; however, a plan must be developed and carried out to maintain long-term adherence to new, healthier habits.

It may be wise, therefore, is to develop the plan so that clients are at least aware of the activities expected to be completed within a 24-hour period. Not surprisingly, however, some clients will adhere to these—or some of these—actions better than others. You cannot mandate a person to maintain a structured day on an hour-by-hour basis. Therefore, it may be best to begin with relatively few rituals—even just one—and increase the number of rituals every couple of weeks or when the client is receptive.

The Importance of Linking the Action Plan to Client Values

As discussed earlier, values consist of core beliefs about what clients feel is important in life and then to incorporate activities—rituals—into their daily schedule that reflect their values as much as possible. For instance, the value of *faith* would be supported by daily prayer. In addition, engaging in regular exercise would reflect the value of health. Values, then, form a strong component of the types of activities that are scheduled in the client's action plan. Remember, too, that there are *costs and consequences* for maintaining improper or unhealthy habits that form the basis for disconnects. Clients sometimes need to be reminded of what those costs and consequences are.

Components of the Time Management Schedule (Action Plan)

The time management schedule should include each of the following areas:

1. *Sleep*: Sleep is a significant factor in maintaining good health, energy and information processing efficiency during the day. More on this topic later. It is important to insert a specific time for "lights out" for sleep and a planned time for awakening. This is because so many people are sleep-deprived. And remember to include presleep rituals that need to be implemented within two hours of bedtime. According to the National Sleep Foundation, TV watching in the bedroom should be avoided, particularly within two hours of sleeping. Their research has found that TV shows, especially in the evening, have violent, arousal-inducing themes and news that impair sleeping. Clients should engage in presleep rituals that prepare the person for peaceful overnight rest, a low heart rate, and reduced body temperature.
2. *Exercise*: Most Western societies include a lifestyle that is far too sedentary. All action plans much include a period for daily vigorous activity. This is especially important because the most frequent excuse given for not exercising is "not enough time." The action plan *must* include designating specific days of the week and time of day for vigorous physical activity. Examples would be formal exercise (e.g., jogging, walking, strength training), recreational activities, and sport participation.
3. *Meals and snacks*: The literature is clear that food is not the enemy. Food provides energy, increases metabolism, and—if consumed strategically—actually helps control weight. Eating habits that produce optimal energy and help control weight consist of consuming several "small" meals per day. This includes three scheduled meals (small portions), interspersed with two snack times, mid-morning and mid-afternoon. Snacks should consist of nutritional, easily digestible foods such as fruit, yogurt, or energy bars. Failure to schedule meals and snacks often results in skipping meals, eating compulsively with unhealthy fast food, or oversnacking. Coaches should refer their clients to a registered dietician to assist clients to make proper food choices.
4. *Recovery breaks*: Inherent in the DVM and consistent with energy management is taking scheduled recovery breaks during the day. I have spoken with hundreds of employees in the corporate sector who are on the go all day without taking a break for proper food and water intake. Then they go home and crash and wonder why they have no energy at night for their family and friends.

The central theme of this work strategy is that "less is more." Humans need time to recover from cognitive and motor demands on the system; it's called "fatigue" in both physical and mental forms. The body needs to completely rest or at least to redirect our focus and concentration every 90–120 minutes, even for just a few minutes. Having a nutritious snack, walking, or engaging in a task that does not require the same type of activity and intensity as the ongoing work task is needed. Schedule it.

5. *Reflect & Plan* (R&P): Our culture seems to reward and recognize people who work hard but fails to recognize the importance of taking the time to reflect and plan. Too often we maintain an impulsive, rather than a reflective, work and thinking pattern. The purpose of R&P is to insert time in our daily schedule for slowing down, reflecting on our day—including the errors (failures) as well as the "home runs" (successes)—and planning tomorrow's goals and activities. This is especially true in our corporate culture. We need to learn from unmet expectations and to appreciate and reinforce our successes. Taking time—even 15–20 minutes—at the end of a workday to think about the days' past events and to plan activities for tomorrow should become a ritual. Educators are another group that requires this strategy.
6. *Making time for family and friends (work-life balance)*: Each of us has developed important relationships with people in our personal life; spouses, parents, siblings, children, neighbors, and others. The time management action plan should include time to connect with these significant others. Sample activities include correspondence (electronic or telephone), personal interaction, and private time for conversation.

   We've all heard the catch phrase "time flies." Weeks and months (sometimes years) pass before we take the time to connect with others. Because personal relationships provide such an important balance in our professional life, we need to create a ritual to "slow down time" and to integrate time for others as part of our week. It's called "work/life balance."
7. *Electronic devices*. Notice that the sample time management sheet includes two sessions for reading and answering e-mail. There is considerable research on the effects of electronic correspondence, such as texting, e-mail, twitter, Facebook, and mobile phone use, on work efficiency and productivity. Much time is wasted sending and answering contacts sent in electronic form. Specific times should be set aside for e-mail correspondence and other electronic devices if productivity is a goal.

Value ——	Sample Value: Health	New Ritual——	Daily brisk walking/resistance training
Value ——	Sample Value: Family	New Ritual——	Get proper rest to maintain energy for family. Spend more time with kids.
Value ——		New Ritual——	
Value ——		New Ritual——	

Sample 24-Hour Time Management Worksheet

4:00 a.m.		4:00 p.m.	**Last meeting or see supervisor**
4:30 a.m.		4:30 p.m.	**Check e-mail/supervisor mtg.**
5:00 a.m.		5:00 p.m.	**Reflect & Plan (for next day)**
5:30 a.m.	**Wake up; wash up**	5:30 p.m.	**Leave for home (or work out)**
6:00 a.m.	**Breakfast (home); feed children**	6:00 p.m.	**Travel or exercise**
6:30 a.m.	**Children to school; read newspaper**	6:30 p.m.	**End workout; home for dinner**
7:00 a.m.	**Leave for work**	7:00 p.m.	**Finish dinnertime with family or time with spouse/partner**
7:30 a.m.	**Travel to work**	7:30 p.m.	**Finish dinner on late exercise days**
8:00 a.m.	**Begin work day; plan day; coffee; review work schedule; e-mail**	8:00 p.m.	**Television or read (no TV watching in bedroom)**
8:30 a.m.	**First appointment**	8:30 p.m.	**During evening social correspondence**
9:00 a.m.		9:00 p.m.	**Leisurely walk**
9:30 a.m.		9:30 p.m.	**Presleep rituals; light snack**
10:00 a.m.	**Take break/snack/walk**	10:00 p.m.	**Personal time**
10:30 a.m.		10:30 p.m.	**Go to sleep**
11:00 a.m.		11:00 p.m.	
11:30 a.m.		11:30 p.m.	
Noon	**Exercise M-W-F Lunch T-Th**	Midnight	
12:30 p.m.	**Exercise or post-lunch walk**	12:30 a.m.	
1:00 p.m.	**End exercise & eat light or begin p.m. schedule (meetings)**	1:00 a.m.	
1:30 p.m.		1:30 a.m.	
2:00 p.m.		2:00 a.m.	
2:30 p.m.		2:30 a.m.	
3:00 p.m.	**Snack and 15-minute recovery break**	3:00 a.m.	
3:30 p.m.		3:30 a.m.	

Required inserted activities: Meals, snacks, sleep, waking up, exercise, recovery breaks

One-Time Action Steps

Starting and maintaining a new, healthier set of habits to replace our old, "bad" routines is very challenging. Sometimes changing an unhealthy habit is facilitated by an "ignition switch"; in this model, it is called a "one-time action step." A one-time action step initiates behavior change by taking "immediate" action prior to or in addition to developing and carrying out a 24-hour time management plan that establishes a time, place, and routine. Perhaps the best way to explain the words "one-time action step" is to think of the word "ignition." An ignition is a "spark," or initiative," in facilitating behavior change. It consists of ways to restart the process of completing our mission toward our goals of better health, success, and quality of life—one step at a time.

As indicated earlier, for both the time management action plan (that builds rituals) and the one-time action plan, it is important to link each new habit to the clients' deepest values—their core beliefs about which they feel passionate and will more likely lead to behavior change. Researchers have found that establishing new long-term (lifestyle) routines, such as regular exercise, drinking more water, presleep rituals, better sleep quality, developing a more rewarding personal life, or changes in eating habits, become automatic in about six to 12 weeks, depending on various personal and environmental factors. Over time, these habits come naturally and are virtually automatic to the client.

However, in order to establish a long-term commitment to health behavior change, we often need a short-term, immediate "spark" to get off the starting blocks to begin the journey toward improved wellness. One-time action steps that consist of planned tasks intended to make an almost immediate impact on the client's quality of life will lead to improved health and wellness.

Here are different types of one-time action steps that expand one's capacity to perform physically (e.g., improved fitness, nutrition, hydration, sleep), mentally (e.g., improved concentration, adapting effectively to life's storms, proper time management), emotionally (e.g., self-control, staying positive, managing negative emotion), and spiritually (e.g., acting in accordance with your values, developing a mission, feeling passionate about what's really important).

Expanding Physical Capacity

One-time action steps to *expand physical capacity* include purchasing a fitness club membership, starting an exercise program (for you and, perhaps, with your spouse, friend, or partner), hiring a personal trainer, consulting a registered dietician to change current eating habits, purchasing a heart rate monitor or new fitness clothing, stocking your office refrigerator with water bottles—drinking about 64 oz. of water per day is recommended by many dieticians—or healthy snacks, registering for a new exercise course, buying a book (or taking one out from the library), making an appointment with an expert to improve your life (physician, clergy member, or mental health professional), or starting new pre-sleep rituals within two hours of bedtime to improve sleep.

Expanding Mental Capacity

Examples of expanding mental capacity include developing a new time management system (e.g., scheduling regular exercise; planning times and content of meals; joining a new club or organization that promotes learning or improved performance; planning daily recovery breaks such as taking a 10- or 15-minute recovery break every 90–120 minutes, such as walking, drinking water, aerobic and strength exercise, brief and nonintrusive socializing).

Guidelines for recovery breaks consist of doing something that the person does not do all day. Recovery may include, for instance, getting away from the computer screen for at least three minutes every 20 minutes (to reduce eye strain), avoiding multitasking (focusing on only one thing at a time), or taking 10–20 minutes to reflect on past accomplishments of the day and planning the rest of the day referred to earlier as "reflect and plan.

Expanding Emotional Capacity

One-time action steps to *expand emotional capacity* may include getting a massage, learning and applying new ways of coping with acute and chronic forms of stress—life's storms—or, to improve one's mood state, using a strategy called "Act as if. . ." Act as if you are feeling good, healthy, positive, and confident. The person's actions remain positive; upbeat; and, at work, always professional even if feelings are unpleasant. Researchers have found that individuals whose actions are positive, friendly, upbeat, and task focused tend to actually feel better and have more positive emotions than a person whose behaviors reflect negative emotions. Thus, if you had a poor night sleep or do not feel energetic, you will feel and perform better if your actions are positive. How we act is more important in determining mood than what we feel; our actions dictate our emotions.

Expanding Spiritual (Values-Based) Capacity

This section concerns one-time activities that are related to the client's passion and values. Activities in this section connect to the client's sense of purpose, or mission, about doing what is personally important in self-growth or in making a difference in the lives of others. Examples of spiritual one-time action steps are attending religious services, contributing to a favorite charity, developing a mission statement, starting "date night" with your spouse or partner, buying your loved one a gift, giving your children more personal time and attention (build this into the daily schedule), volunteering for community or job-related service, finding a mentor, mentoring another person, leaving family members a weekly note to say "I love you," daily prayer, and acknowledging one's deepest values *and* holding oneself accountable to them each day. Family and friends take precedence in determining one-time action steps.

One-time action plans are about finding ways to confirm the person's commitment to "getting started" by making short-term, rapid, and relevant steps toward a better, more satisfying, and healthier life and lifestyle. Taking one or more immediate steps reflects one's commitment to changing one or more behaviors until the longer-term action plan kicks in. The result will be more (higher quality) years remaining to love family, have more energy, be more productive, and to be available to those who love and need you. The following table allows the client to insert his/her own one-time action steps.

Client One-Time Action Steps	Starting Date
Insert: (a) Category of expansion (physical, mental, emotional, or values-based); (b) the specific activity; and (c) the starting date for that planned action.	
Sample: (a) Expand physical capacity; (b) meet with a performance coach to start new exercise program.	**Monday, January 26, 2016**
1.	
2.	
3.	
4.	
5.	
6.	
7.	
8.	
9.	

Concluding Issues about the Action Plan

As indicated earlier, the action plan is not the final segment of the health behavior change process (according to the DVM). The *final* segment consists of carrying out cognitive and behavioral strategies that promote adherence to the client's new rituals, material covered in Part 4, chapters 12–14. These new rituals serve the purpose of ensuring that the client's habits are consistent with his or her core beliefs and values. The importance of developing the client's action plan, including one-time action steps, rests on the need to specify and schedule future activities that are life-changing and will improve the client's health, energy, and quality of life.

The Problem of Overprescribing Strategies

Therapists and coaches must be warned about a behavior pattern called *overprescribing*. The therapist's/coach's eagerness to provide clients with helpful guidance and successful outcomes may result in prescribing too many cognitive and/or behavioral strategies for the client to handle and apply properly. Take goal setting, for example. Clients may be asked to set short-term goals, long-term goals, process-oriented (performance) goals, and product-oriented (outcome) goals. This "requirement" is in addition to following other goal-setting strategies, such as keeping goals challenging but achievable, measurable, and linked to previous performance level. Adding the use of other mental skills and cognitive strategies such as mental imagery, positive self-talk, anticipation, association, dissociation, psyching up, and others can confuse and befuddle clients. What was intended to be performance-enhancing and effective techniques can become intrusive, confusing, and frustrating, resulting in diminishing returns.

A related potential problem in the prescribing area is to ask clients to make too many sudden changes to their daily routines. For example, while committing to a new exercise program is laudable, combining a change in one ritual—exercise—(practiced several times a week) with other, new rituals—let's say avoiding meals within an hour or two of bedtime, developing new presleep rituals, and learning new coping strategies in response to stressful experiences during the day—is overreaching. Mental health professionals, by their nature, personality, and training, want to help others achieve as many desirable goals as possible. In their haste to provide valuable and effective service to clients, some consultants will simply overprescribe. This explains the cliché "a little knowledge can be dangerous."

The preferred counseling/coaching strategy is to teach clients to carry out one strategy at a time then repeat it until it's practiced almost automatically. That is what makes it a ritual. After "ritual A" has been achieved and mastered, then "ritual B" can be introduced to the client. All rituals should be connected to at least one of the client's values.

How long does it take to automate a ritual? The answer to this question differs from study to study, but the common wisdom is that the length of time needed to learn and apply a new ritual depends on the ritual's complexity, is a reflection of the client's personality and connection to other individuals and environmental conditions, and is linked to the client's previous experiences with the ritual. Former athletes, for instance, are more likely to adopt an exercise routine more quickly than exercise novices—clients who have never engaged in regular exercise outside of their school PE classes. Former athletes or retired military also have the tendency to be more disciplined and willing to carry out instructions than persons who have never been subjected to performing under harsh conditions or in accordance with detailed schedules on which building new rituals rely.

One more issue about developing and carrying an action plan concerns the coach's willingness to monitor the client's progress. This is becoming common practice in the health insurance industry in recent years in which a "health coach" (or similar title) establishes contact during the client's (patient's) membership year to ask if the client has any health-related questions, needs assistance from a fitness or nutrition coach, or ensures that the client is adhering to predetermined tasks and remaining on track to meet goals.

Another example comes from the sleep clinic industry, which tests individuals for a variety of sleep illnesses, most notably sleep apnea—the cessation of breathing during sleep or the obstruction of the patient's airways, which can lead to a heart attack (myocardial infarction) or stroke. Patients with sleep apnea are given the opportunity or, in severe cases, urged, to use a device that forces air through the patient's nostrils using a CPAP machine (Continuous Positive Airway Pressure). Health insurance will pay for the machine *only if* the client uses it a minimum of four hours per 24-hour period. Two sources of coaching, the sleep clinic and the CPAP machine distributor, have contact with the patient via a personal office visit and over the phone during the first 90 days of machine use to help ensure client compliance. Remediation to improve CPAP compliance is offered regularly, but patients may seek assistance at any time. Consistent use of this machine is potentially lifesaving and certainly, at the very least, health enhancing. See Rotech Healthcare Inc. at www.rotech.com for further information about this device.

The suggestion in applying the DVM's action plan is to start slow, install the new routine that is easiest and in which the client is most motivated to begin and maintain, be sure the client is offered coaching or social support to assure compliance with the ritual, and monitor client progress. Finally, it is suggested that coaches/therapists measure change in client progress, which requires recording preintervention (baseline) scores and then retesting six to 10 weeks later to (hopefully) detect improvement in outcomes. Numbers, such as test data, often motivates behavior.

Mental Skills that Promote Exercise Performance

A coach/therapist uses any of these skills prior to and during a client's exercise regimen.

Your thoughts influence emotions, mood, effort, and exercise performance. Here are suggestions taken from the exercise psychology literature that help promote exercise performance and performance outcomes. These mental skills are divided into two components, pre-exercise skills (performed prior to a formal exercise session) and exercise-related skills (performed with the exercise activity).

I. Pre-Exercise Mental Skills

1. **Develop an exercise routine; schedule it.** Ultimately, the goal of any exerciser is to ritualize his or her fitness program. Researchers claim that we thrive on rituals because they help reduce stress, cut down on the number

of things we have to plan and think about, and promote overall well-being. An exercise ritual—scheduling our exercise times and locations—reduces the chance of "forgetting" or running out of time to exercise.

2. **Positive Self-Talk (pre-exercise thoughts).** Have you ever said to yourself, before attending a fitness facility or before exercising, "I don't want to do this," or "Do I really have to exercise today?" What about the content of your thoughts during exercise? Positive (e.g., "I can do this"; "I feel good") or negative (e.g., "I am not enjoying this," or "This really sucks")? Studies show that the content of your thinking—positive or negative—influences performance.
3. **Develop a positive attitude and self-confidence toward exercise.** The enthusiasm you feel toward any task or program will result in better adherence and superior outcomes. See the "big picture" about the benefits—short term and long term—of your involvement, and be committed to experience the full program. Do not let others or one or two individual experiences control your destiny. This is your health and quality of life we are talking about. Feel confident in your ability to learn and improve, and expect to receive all the benefits you deserve from the energy you are investing in this program. Along these lines, remember to live a life that is consistent with your values (e.g., health, family, high-quality job performance, faith, excellence, and so on).
4. **Have realistic but challenging performance (not outcome) goals.** The extensive research on goal setting is clear; goals tend to increase motivation; help the performer focus his or her energy toward the desired outcome; and fulfill a personal need to achieve and to feel competent, both of which are normal and desirable. To have goals that are credible, however, be sure your goals are challenging but not unrealistic. Although a few beginning exercisers decide to train for eventually running a marathon (i.e., a 26-mile race), this is not realistic thinking for most of us.

   A sample outcome goal is "I will finish in first or second place in the race" or "I will lose 10 pounds by the end of next month." Performance goal examples, which are especially important, are "I will be able to lift two 25-pound dumb bells for 10 repetitions by the end of this month" or "I will be able to jog/run around the track nonstop within three minutes."
5. **Receive proper instruction and coaching.** Exercise is a science; there is a right way and a wrong way to perform exercises and improve cardio and strength fitness. Listen to your fitness coach and ask questions. This is a crucial strategy in getting fit and reaching your goals. Invest in your health and work with a fitness coach for at least four or five sessions. Know how to exercise properly and obtain baseline results of your fitness level. Try to read publications—books, journals, articles—that provide science-based information about proper exercise techniques. In addition, your program or fitness coach will (should) discuss these with you.

6. **Obtain fitness tests.** Humans thrive on data—numbers from test results—which motivate us to change behavior. Ask any doctor about the best motivator to change a patient's unhealthy habits. Fitness testing also provides your coach with direction to provide an accurate exercise prescription.

II. Exercise-Related Mental Skills

1. **Positive self-talk.** Although discussed earlier with respect to pre-exercise thinking, this is a strategy that is essential to good exercise performance. Before your exercise session, be optimistic about the likely outcomes of your exercise session and of your involvement in the program; equally important, think "upbeat" thoughts *during* your exercise session. Your energy level—and, hence, exercise performance—will actually improve in response to positive self-talk, as opposed to having negative thoughts.
2. **Association.** Association refers to connecting one's thoughts to bodily sensations, that is, focusing on specific body parts and muscle groups during exertion. Thus, when lifting weights, the exerciser uses association by focusing his or her attention on the muscles most heavily involved in that lift. When performing a bicep curl, for example, exercisers would focus their attention on the bicep muscle primarily responsible for that action. In response to cardiovascular activity, runners use association to think about the bodily sensations during the run—connecting thoughts to actions. Less fit folks prefer to *not use* association during cardiovascular exercise because those thoughts are not always pleasant. Instead, they would use dissociation.
3. **Dissociation.** Instead of focusing on the muscles being used or the bodily sensations being experienced during exercise, dissociation is concerned with disconnecting one's mind with one's exertion. The use of music when performing physical activity, especially when exercise is performed in synchronization to music, is a good example of a dissociation strategy. The person is focusing his or her attention on external stimuli rather than on bodily sensations experienced during exercise. Dissociation is a common technique used during cardiovascular work, but not weight training, in which your attentional focus should be on the muscle group being exerted.
4. **Bizarre imagery.** This strategy concerns thinking about the impossible. Imagery concerns visualizing an action, that is, a mental representation of actual performance. *Bizarre* imagery means that the thought content cannot occur in reality yet is motivational to the performer. Examples include thinking about "washing away" plaque against the walls of arteries or having your fat "melt away" when performing aerobic activity. Cancer patients have used bizarre imagery to image shrinking tumors when receiving chemotherapy.
5. **Music.** Have you ever participated in an aerobics class in which you were moving to music—and felt more energy than when exercising in the absence of music? Music is a distractor, helping the person focus on external (musical)

stimuli, while the person gives minimal attention to bodily sensations associated with physical effort (e.g., fatigue, sweating, exertion, high heart rate, discomfort). Exercising with fast-paced music tends to increase arousal level, which allows the person to move with greater intensity. Slower-paced music reduces arousal and heart rate, which is sometimes desirable. Slower rhythms improve relaxation and lower heart rate.

6. **Social support.** If you like to exercise with a friend or receive recognition from friends, family, or colleagues, you are experiencing social support. Support is one of the leading predictors of exercise adherence—after beginning an exercise program, you stay with it. Social support can be direct (e.g., exercising with another person or receiving instruction or coaching) or indirect (e.g., others offer praise, recognition, or approval without exercising with you). Some individuals, however, prefer to exercise alone or do not find it motivating to receive attention from others.
7. **Psyching up.** The goal here is to improve arousal level, excitation, or positive emotion, which, in turn, increases effort and physical exertion. Examples of psyching-up strategies can be verbal (e.g., "Come on, I can do this"; "go for it"; "Let's get this done"; "Do it, do it, do it") or nonverbal (e.g., increasing exertion during a particular phase of an exercise, perhaps when lifting weights).

In summary, mental skills are often ignored or not known to exercisers yet have an important role in improving exercise performance. There is a strong link between the mind and body, and what you think (also called cognition) and feel (emotion) will directly influence your physical performance. Many of these strategies are used by world-class athletes as part of their training and during competition.

Exercise Adherence Strategies for Overcoming Exercise Barriers

Exercise barriers are inherent to starting and maintaining any new healthy habit—exercise, improved nutrition, coping with stress, and taking recovery breaks, to name a few. Here is some information on ways to combat barriers to the program's number one goal—adhering to your new exercise program. Each of these barriers, although real, is controllable and, therefore, can be managed, according to the research exercise psychology literature.

Not Enough Time: Without question, this is the most common explanation for not exercising—or dropping out after starting a fitness program. Is it realistic? Can we actually run out of time? Answers: (a) The excuse of "no time" is a perception—a person's subjective view of things. It may or may not have anything to do with reality. (b) There are 168 hours in a week. If we exercised just three of those hours, which is the minimum that researchers suggest, that would be only ONE PERCENT of our total week (3 of 168). (c) Exercise is an investment; a bit less time now to do other things, but much more time to do things later and more efficiently due to more energy. Not enough time? We spend 10% of our week in front of the TV and 5–6% on the phone. What's your priority when it comes to good health? How about waking up an hour early twice a week for an early-morning exercise bout? Perhaps come home one hour later twice a week due to your exercise routine after work.

Lack of fitness information/knowledge: This is a very common problem because no one teaches most of us how to exercise correctly. Consequently, our poor form results in discomfort, injury, and lack of effective results. That's why this program has coaching—a lot of it (e.g., fitness, nutrition, mental health, work related). I also invite you to purchase written materials on fitness, Be your own coach or hire a personal trainer.

Lack of confidence: This comes with improvement, mastery of exercise skills (such as weight training and proper use of the machines), and the perception of competence. Most successful people have a personality trait called high need achievement. We place ourselves in achievement settings, set challenging goals, and have high self-expectations toward achieving those goals. Therefore, it is natural to feel low confidence (and, therefore, be uncomfortable) in settings in which we are novices or relatively unskilled. As you gain experience and progress in your exercise skills and fitness level, your confidence will increase—dramatically. Confidence is all about task mastery, so stay the course!

Intimidated to exercise in public: Some individuals are self-conscious and embarrassed to exercise in a public setting. Why is this and what can they do about it?" First, most people are too busy exercising to pay attention to you Second, stop caring what other people think. Stop empowering others to dictate your behavior. Third, the best way to stop thinking about what others think is to develop routines upon entering the exercise venue and keep moving. No need to stop and look around, unless you feel comfortable making eye contact. Working out with a friend is one way to focus on the task at hand and avoid intimidation.

Do not have an exercise partner: Your fitness coach can help you, here Tell your fitness coach you are looking for someone with whom to exercise. Your coach will ask around for others who exercise at a similar time and are also happy to work out with a partner. You can also invite your partner (spouse, friend) or work colleague to exercise with you.

Lack of support from partner and others: Is your partner sabotaging or inhibiting your attempts to exercise regularly? You don't want your desire to get fit, lose weight, and become healthier to cause a divorce. You want your partner to support you, not to become jealous of your attempts to lose weight and become healthier." Insecurity does nasty things to people's minds. First and foremost, try to include your partner in your exercise routine. Second, try exercising at home—again, with your partner, if possible. Third, try to exercise during the day when at work rather than leaving the house early or coming home late due to your exercise routine. If all else fails, then work with a professional counselor to determine the reasons your partner or family will not support your wish to exercise. Bottom line is this: healthy relationships are based on supporting your partner, especially when it comes to improving one's health. If someone does not want you to exercise, seek professional help to find out the reason(s) and change the situation.

History of giving up: This is amazingly common. So many people say, "I tend to stop what I start, so why even try?" Or they will quit exercising when they are forced to temporarily stop, perhaps due to illness, vacation, or injury (a phenomenon called the "abstinence relapse effect"). Your body will "retrain" quickly after stopping temporarily. Do not give up. Also, having an exercise partner, hiring a personal trainer, setting goals, meeting social needs, exercising in a comfortable venue (even home), and detecting progress are all ways in which a person can feel reinforced and positive about his or her exercise participation.

Too expensive (e.g., exercise clothing, personal trainer, club membership): Exercise clothing and equipment make great gifts, so ask for something that will promote your exercise habit. Or save up a few dollars, buy one less new outfit, or take a few extra dollars from that next paycheck and treat yourself well. Do all that you can to support your new exercise habit.

Not close access to exercise facility: Researchers have found that people will not travel more than about three blocks out of their way between work and home to attend an exercise facility. If this is your situation, try to exercise at work (if not in a fitness facility, then walk stairs, walk across part of campus, do sit-ups in your office, ANYTHING that causes you to move), or buy exercise equipment for your home. The reason we tend to ignore our home exercise equipment is because we lack structured routines to use it. In addition, we tend to think of home as a place to relax and spend our time with passive entertainment devices, eating, speaking on the phone—anything but exercise. Equipment collects dust—our promises and New Year's Eve resolutions to the contrary.

Fear of injury: This fear is not at all uncommon, especially as we age and have a few aches, pains, and previous surgeries and illnesses. So, with assistance from your physician, personal trainer, and, perhaps a physical therapist, exercise intelligently. Be sure to be aware of your physical limitations, but do not avoid vigorous physical activity. Your muscles—including your heart, which is a muscle—need it.

Find exercise unpleasant: Bottom line is that many of us just dislike exercising. Of course, we have trained ourselves to be sedentary, so exercise—which we all KNOW is good for our health—is stressful and unpleasant. "You are who you train to be!" Some of us can also blame our former physical education teachers and sports coaches who made us exercise as a form of punishment (where we started associating exercise with bad behavior, making exercise something to avoid) and a culture of laziness. We do not enjoy moving our bodies. But as we age, we begin paying a heavy price for our sedentary lifestyle. Disease, malfunctioning body parts, and low energy start to become more obvious. We begin to pay the price, which can be seen in our poorer health, diminished happiness, reduced work productivity, and lower quality of life. Become enthusiastic about developing healthy rituals, including exercise. You cannot be both enthusiastic and unhappy at the same time.

References

Anshel, M.H. (2014). *Applied health fitness psychology*. Champaign, IL: Human Kinetics.

Loehr, J., & Schwartz, T. (2003). *The power of full engagement: Managing energy, not time, is the key to high performance and personal renewal*. New York: The Free Press.

Segar, M.L., Eccles, J.S., & Richardson, C.R. (2011). Rebranding exercise: closing the gap between values and behavior. *International Journal of Behavioral Nutrition and Physical Activity*, *8*, pp. 94–108.

PART IV

Adherence and Compliance to New Healthy Habits

12

ADHERENCE AND COMPLIANCE TO HEALTHY HABITS

Not finishing what we start is a common habit. It's called "quitting," "dropping out," or what researchers and practitioners label "nonadherence" or "noncompliance." Why, then, do so many of us begin a program or change a habit and then revert back to our previous ways of doing things? Why do we "drop the ball," and what can health professionals do about it? The focus of this chapter is to address a person's decision to maintain new, healthy habits. The concept of *adherence*, and its "sister" concept *compliance*, need to be defined and clarified. This is important because the process of building a habit/ritual reflects success of the DVM program and action plan with respect to short-term and long-term maintenance of any lifestyle change. Is the client still engaged in the same ritual(s) and has it become a permanent change in behavior?

Defining Adherence and Compliance

Defining adherence has differed from study to study in the area of health. In addition, some authors no longer distinguish between *adherence* and *compliance*, which has become increasingly neglected in recent years. King (1994) defines *adherence* as "the level of participation achieved in a behavioral regimen once the individual has agreed to undertake it" (p. 186). *Compliance* is a term often used interchangeably, but incorrectly, with adherence. Many writers, however, contend these two concepts are distinctly different. Compliance is often defined as "the degree to which an individual follows a specific recommendation" (Bowen, Helmes, & Lease, 2001, p. 26) or "the extent to which a person's behavior (in terms of taking medication, following a diet, modifying habits [such as exercise], or attending clinics) coincides with medical or health advise" (Haynes, 2001, p. 4).

Haynes points out that the term "adherence" (rather than compliance) is preferred because compliance, he believes, "implies subservience on the part of the patient, or constitutes blaming the patient for noncompliance" (p. 4). Thus, adherence is a concept that reflects individuals' *self-determined action*, that is, their own decision to maintain participation in an exercise program that they selected based on their own volition, while compliance reflects the decision to maintain participation in a program that was prescribed or required by others. Nonadherence is a function of one's own decision to terminate involvement in an activity, while noncompliance consists of acting in a manner that is contrary to advice or one's recommendations or requirements (i.e., I will not take—or continue to take—the medication my doctor prescribed).

Rand and Weeks (1998) define the terms adherence and compliance interchangeably "as the degree to which patient behaviors coincide with the clinical recommendations of health care providers" (p. 115). This definition is more closely linked to the traditional definition of compliance, whereas adherence is a self-determined decision in which the person decides to exercise on his or her own volition in the absence of being prompted or required by someone else to exercise. Rand and Weeks claim that there is no clear description of adherence to health behaviors labeled "satisfactory" or "poor." They assert that appropriate adherence must be operationally (situationally) defined based on the situation and desired outcomes. For instance, taking a certain medication or carrying out a preoperation regimen at home might be very challenging if the required set of actions requires extensive preparation. Engaging in certain types of exercise at specific times of the day for physical rehabilitation is another example of defining compliance operationally (specific to the situation). Here, then, are the recognized formal definitions of compliance and adherence:

Compliance: A physician or personal trainer prescribes a specific exercise routine to an individual who then follows that prescription. A client follows the diet and/or nutritional advice prescribed by a registered dietician. In both examples, the prescription is based on patient (client) test data.

Adherence: The client/patient initiates and maintains an exercise routine that is communicated by a specialist and is intended to meet the client's/patient's needs (e.g., lose weight, improve lipids profile) and reach predetermined goals (e.g., improved aerobic fitness, increase high-density cholesterol).

Types of Adherence and Compliance

As indicated earlier, clinicians and researchers agree that adherence and compliance have multiple dimensions and definitions. Adherence often categorizes individuals as "adherers" ("compliers") or "nonadherers" ("noncompliers"). Adherence, however, is not a dichotomous variable (e.g., "yes–no;" "good–poor"). Unlike the concept of a "dropout" or "nonparticipant," which *is* a "yes" or "no" variable, adherence rarely reflects a person who did or did not adhere to the researcher's or clinician's expectations. Thus, adherence is often computed and determined as a matter of degree and must be situationally defined. In their review of literature, for instance, Rand and Weeks (1998) categorize adherence according to the extent to which a person engages in the targeted (criterion) task. Here are subcategories of adherence.

"Appropriate" adherence. Refers to a patient, client, or participant who performs "expected" behavior over time. A person asked to consume several small meals per day instead of skipping some meals or eating excessively at mealtime will carry out that prescribed dietary regimen daily.

Erratic adherence. Also called *partial compliance*, a person follows a prescribed program or takes medication as required some days/weeks but must withdraw or change the prescribed/required behavior other times. For instance, certain activities are necessary in the presence of certain symptoms (e.g., the use of antihistamines during allergy season, antibiotics following a surgical procedure, or a stretching protocol in response to an injury) but are no longer needed when the symptoms are no longer detected. As Rand and Weeks (1998) contend, "erratic adherence may also reflect forgetfulness, stress, changed schedules . . . or some other barriers to full adherence" (p. 116).

Noncompliance. Reflects a person's chronic underuse of a substance or treatment. Thus, an individual who is asked but fails to complete and a series of nightly presleep rituals to obtain a better night sleep will fulfill this requirement.

Erratic noncompliance. This behavior is characterized by the individual's perceptions and behaviors of being too busy, forgetful, or stressed or experiencing some acute problem.

Unwitting noncompliance. This form of not completing a prescribed or expected protocol might include misunderstanding the task or instructions, incorrect use of proper techniques (e.g., proper use of their CPAP machine to obtain a better night sleep), inability to travel to receive treatment, experiencing injury or pain, or lack of social support.

Intentional noncompliance. Indicative of improved well-being, fear of injury or reoccurring symptoms, a dislike of exercising, refusal to adapt to a new lifestyle, physical or psychological discomfort from exercise, or denial of exercise benefits.

Measuring Adherence

It is apparent that persons who agree to engage in a given activity and then discontinue their involvement in that same activity are not adhering. Sadly, this is an all-too-common problem in the area of health behavior. People often do not finish what they start; program maintenance is a concern in the medical and health community. However, the determination of adherence and compliance (or nonadherence and noncompliance, respectively) often differs among studies. Do we consider a person an exercise dropout if he or she were prescribed a cardiovascular fitness program based on three 30-minute sessions per week but can attend only twice per week? Or is the use of medical equipment (e.g., a CPAP machine to reduce sleep apnea, rehabilitation exercise equipment, nicotine patch to reduce the urge to smoke) adherence if the person completes only a segment of the prescribed treatment? Certainly, the motives and explanations for not completing an intervention are different, depending on the reasons and both situational and personal factors. If people quit their treatment due to boredom or laziness, that reflects an issue that requires one type of reaction by a health professional. A different adherence strategy is warranted if the person fails to complete treatment due to a factor beyond his or her control, such as an illness, injury, lack of transportation, bad weather, equipment malfunction, and lack of proper coaching, among other possible reasons. Haynes (2001) recommends using three means to detect adherence:

(1) *Appointment attendance*: Assuming there is a planned program at which the participant is expected to attend, Haynes suggests watching for individuals who fail to attend prearranged appointments or programs. In addition, individuals who are partial, or irregular, attendees are less likely to be adhering to their program.
(2) *Detecting nonresponders*: Nonadherence is the most frequent explanation for lack of improved fitness or any other expected and desirable outcome. It is also important, however, to be sure that the individual is engaging in the proper exercise procedures under the most desirable conditions (e.g., using the correct resistance in weight training, running/walking according to a prescribed plan, feeling comfortable and motivated during exercise, having adequate water before and during exercise).
(3) *Asking nonresponders about their adherence*: It is appropriate to simply ask individuals if they are attending exercise sessions and following through on their planned program—diet, exercise, rehabilitation—in the prescribed manner. This procedure, however, has to be carried out in a very nonthreatening, sensitive manner so that the individual does not feel defensive or become insecure or anxious about speaking the "truth."

Other measures of adherence. Adherence can also be ascertained by using the following options: (a) attendance at predetermined events (e.g., exercise class, appointments, meetings); (b) self-reporting (i.e., the person indicates his or her own adherence to the program); (c) record keeping, in which the person completes an attendance chart; (d) monitoring progress (e.g., changes in resting heart rate, body weight, running speed, endurance time, or body weight), (e) testing (e.g., lipids profile, aerobic or strength fitness testing); (f) number of contacts with staff/coaches; (g) number of appointments kept; (h) interviews with others with whom the person usually keeps in contact (e.g., peers, family members, other professionals, other program attendees); and (i) electronic methods, including the use of computers (Internet), iPods, modems, text messaging, and other electronic means of recording behavior. Pedometers (recording step counts), accelerometers (recording step counts and speed), and heart rate monitors also fall into the category of physical devices that have been studied to influence exercise behavior.

Chenoweth (2007) coined the term *e-health technology* to reflect the phenomenon of using the Internet as a source of health information and behavior. He defines e-health technology as "the application of Internet and other related technologies to improve the access, efficiency, effectiveness, and quality of clinical and business practices used by organizations, practitioners, and consumers to improve and maintain the health status of individuals and organizations" (p. 97).

Applying electronic devices to promote fitness. The proliferation of electronic devices has prompted practitioners to examine the effects of these devices on health behavior, particularly with respect to adherence. Patients are reminded, or prompted, to initiate their healthy habits through texting, phone calls, modems, or computer software, particularly if the communication source is a specialist or expert in a given health area.

Results of several recent studies are promising in improving adherence rates. For instance, Lombard et al. (1995) found that persons who received weekly phone calls to "touch base" walked more often than individuals who were called once every three weeks or not called at all. Phone calls, they concluded, form a source of emotional and social support and hold the individual accountable to his or her earlier agreement to exercise regularly.

In summary, it is important to determine if clients/patients/participants continue to follow through on their new rituals embedded in their action plan. Failure to maintain participation in their program may signal a deficiency in the program's content or the manner in which it is organized or taught and may indicate that more effort is required to follow up with participants on program content; more support is needed during the postprogram (follow-up) phase. On the other hand, the participant's adherence to program content signals program effectiveness, a favorable attitude toward carrying out new healthy routines, and a possible marketing tool in "selling" the program to others.

References

Bowen, D.J., Helmes, A., & Lease, E. (2001). Predicting compliance: How are we doing? In L. E. Burke & I.S. Ockene (Eds.), *Compliance in healthcare and research* (pp. 25–41). Armonk, NY: Futura.

Chenoweth, D.H. (2007). *Worksite health promotion* (2nd ed.). Champaign, IL: Human Kinetics.

Haynes, R.B. (2001). Improving patient adherence: State of the art, with a special focus on Medication-taking for cardiovascular disorders. In L.E. Burke & I.S. Ockene (Eds.), *Compliance in healthcare and research* (pp. 3–21). Armonk, NY: Futura.

King, A.C. (1994). Clinical and community interventions to promote and support physical activity participation. In R.K. Dishman (Ed.), *Advances in exercise psychology* (pp. 183–212). Champaign, IL: Human Kinetics.

Lombard, D.N., Lombard, T.N., & Winnett, R.A. (1995). Walking to meet health guidelines: The effect of prompting frequency and prompt structure. *Health Psychology, 14*, 164–170.

Rand, C.S., & Weeks, K. (1998). Measuring adherence with medication regiments in clinical care and research. In S.A. Shumaker, E.B. Schron, J.K. Ockene, & W.L. Mcbee (Eds.), *The handbook of health behavior change* (2nd ed., pp. 114–132). New York: Springer.

13

STEPS FOR ACHIEVING ADHERENCE TO NEW (HEALTHY) HABITS

Barriers are perceptions; they reflect a person's own belief about the reason a habit cannot be carried out. Barriers also predict whether people will carry out actions that are intended to improve health and manage disease. Health professionals want to help people improve their health by reducing the number of reasons for maintaining unhealthy habits. Every undesirable/unhealthy habit has benefits to the individual or else he or she would not continue to practice it.

The typical barriers for maintaining unhealthy habits, using exercise as an example, include "not enough time," "no one will exercise with me" (lack of social support), "it's too expensive" (e.g., club membership, footwear and clothing purchases), "it is too difficult," I'm not in good shape," and "I'm overweight and need to first lose a few pounds," and "I have leg pain and can only exercise on a bike or in the water." Related explanations that may be classified as irrational thinking include "My whole family is overweight/obese," "My doctor says my health is fine," and (particularly in some cultures more than others) "My health is all in the Lord's hands." These reasons offered for not developing an exercise habit may or may not be accurate and reflect reality. Given the high number of people in many countries who are overweight and obese, made worse by a sedentary lifestyle, high stress, and poor eating and sleeping habits, it is understandable that researchers have found no shortage of reasons why people report they do not engage in regular exercise or stop exercising after initiating an exercise routine. Barriers exist for many other unhealthy habits, as well.

Barriers have been categorized as either objective (e.g., inaccessible facilities for physically disabled persons, disease, injury, lack of an available exercise facility, lack of transportation) or perceived (e.g., lack of time, high cost of a fitness club membership, feeling stress or anxiety about exercising in a public setting or upon entering an exercise facility, avoidance of exertion). Barriers have also been categorized as internal, interpersonal, and environmental (Timmerman, 2007).

Personal barriers include physical fatigue, feeling discomfort, or having family responsibilities that affect one's health and happiness. Personal barriers are associated with a reduced likelihood of building healthy habits into one's schedule and continued unhealthy habits (e.g. less physical activity, excessive TV watching, food consumption close to bedtime, poor sleep). Attempts to reduce dropping out of exercise programs and increasing physical activity, while promoting adherence to new health rituals, require examining the reasons, or motives, for engaging in a new healthy routine. Let's take exercise as one example.

There are numerous reasons people like to exercise or engage in other forms of physical activity. These include, based on the Exercise Motivation Inventory (Markland & Ingledew, 1997), stress management (e.g., "to release tension"), weight management ("to stay slim"), revitalization ("because it makes me feel good"), social recognition ("to gain recognition for my accomplishments"), enjoyment ("because I enjoy the feeling of exerting myself"), challenge ("to help me explore the limits of my body"), social affiliation ("to meet or spend time with friends"), competition ("because I enjoy competing"), health pressures ("my doctor advised me to exercise"), avoiding poor health ("to avoid heart disease or other diseases"), positive health ("to help me live a longer, healthier life"), and appearance ("to have a good body and a nice appearance"). Therefore, given this extensive list of reasons for exercising, the next issue is why stop? What happened to the person's motivation to maintain an exercise habit? These "reasons" for not starting or dropping out of an exercise habit are called *exercise barriers*.

Most studies that list perceived barriers to starting and maintaining healthy habits, especially with respect to exercise, have included lack of time (usually the leading cause in most studies); experiencing pain/discomfort/injury; fear of injury; unavailable exercise equipment or facility; lack of knowledge about proper exercise technique; finding exercise unpleasant; lack of confidence; feeling intimidated; no exercise partner; lack of support from partner/others; a history of giving up, so why start in the first place; too expensive; and no close access to a facility (Brinthaupt, Kang & Anshel, 2010; Buckworth & Dishman, 1999; Lox et al., 2014).

Lack of time. The most common psycho-behavioral exercise barrier reported in the research literature, not surprisingly, is lack of time. In their review of this literature, Brinthaupt et al. (2010) concluded that lack of time is one of the most difficult barriers to overcome. The authors refer to lack of time as a "superbarrier" in that it impacts many other factors related to exercise. For example, lack of time goes beyond actual exercise time. It also may include time and distance for travel to and from an exercise facility or location; time needed (but lost) to perform other valued activities related to work, leisure, family, and hobbies; and time needed to conduct other daily routines that require changing one's personal schedule (Kruger, Yore, Bauer, & Kohl, 2007).

Lack of time is also cited in relation to sources of job stress and ways to manage stress based on maintaining healthy habits. For example, many people who are aware of the need to exercise and eat nutritionally also report that their schedule will "not allow" for engaging in a regular exercise habit; "there is too much work to do," they report. There is a very effective retort to the challenge of perceived insufficient time, which will be addressed later. At this time, however, coaches and therapists should know that enjoying the benefits of exercise consumes only 1.5% of someone's work week.

Discomfort and lack of enjoyment. Another common exercise barrier is a person's discomfort and lack of enjoyment while experiencing high physical exertion, particularly if the exerciser is overweight/obese, inexperienced in executing proper exercise technique, or does not enjoy physical exertion and becoming physically fatigued (Salmon et al., 2003). An unpleasant exercise environment—perhaps an intimidating fitness club or jogging/walking on the street—forms an additional reason to avoid exercise. The goal of every practitioner in the areas of health, fitness, and mental health is to reduce the frequency and intensity of these barriers in overcoming exercise barriers. This is accomplished, at least in part, by helping clients to initiate and maintain a regimen, or schedule, of regular exercise or any other healthy habit for the purpose of developing an active, healthy lifestyle. As indicated earlier, the process. The process by which an individual maintains participation in a preplanned exercise program is called *exercise adherence.*

In summary, determining adherence/nonadherence rates are important to: (a) explain results of interventions, in which the client/patient did not improve on some measure perhaps due to low adherence rates; (b) change intervention content to improve adherence rates (perhaps the prescribed activity was too difficult or did not take certain factors into account, such as transportation, program costs, use of proper equipment, or health status of participants); and (c) determine treatment effects over time, both short term (e.g., during the treatment period or within 60 days after the program) and long term (e.g., more than 60 days, perhaps six months or a year after the program).

Mental Barriers to Adherence

While there are many physical barriers to adhering to a new healthy habit ritual, there are also psychological reasons.

Anxiety. Anxiety is usually defined as a person who has feelings of worry or threat about the future, which is common when trying to initiate a new healthy habit. Exercise settings, for instance, often create anxiety for novice exercisers who lack confidence, are often self-conscious about their appearance, and are concerned about performing exercises correctly and with meeting performance goals. Sources of anxiety include concern about meeting fitness or weight reduction goals; one's physical appearance; developing a sense of belonging in exercise facilities; and using time to exercise instead of doing something else, such as

"I could be finishing a report (watching TV) instead of going to the gym." Interestingly, exercise has been used to reduce both short-term (acute) and long-term (chronic) forms of anxiety. Anxiety may accompany any attempt to learn, integrate, and carry out a new habit that will improve health.

Unrealistically high self-expectations. Too many people quit carrying out their new habit due to having unrealistic expectations (e.g., losing 20 pounds in a month, reducing stress immediately, being able to keep up with the fitness instructor after two weeks of working out, eliminating excessive fat from the tummy or thighs) or starting and carrying out a new daily schedule that integrates several new routines—all at once and starting "today." New rituals have to be introduced one at a time and slowly integrated into one's lifestyle. Nothing should be rushed unless it's a life-threatening issue.

Low perceived competence. We live in a high-pressure, immediate gratification culture filled with unrealistic expectations. It's quite rare for us to persist at any task in which we perform poorly or fail to improve. Conversely, we are attracted to tasks at which we feel competent, improve our performance, and feel more comfortable and confident. To promote exercise adherence, for instance, it is essential to learn the proper exercise techniques, obtain positive feedback on performance, and see positive results from exercise performance—soon. Hiring a personal trainer who will provide the proper exercise prescription and instruction is a good investment for many individuals until they learn to carry out the program independently. Ditto for learning and carrying out any new habit. Working with a specialist or health professional—mental, physical, or medical—is strongly suggested to overcome low perceived competence.

Negative self-talk. Negative self-talk is the process by which an individual engages in a covert monologue consisting of unpleasant feelings. It is virtually impossible for individuals to remain motivated and to concentrate on the task at hand if they are engaging in negative self-talk, especially just prior to or during the process of learning and executing a new habit. Negative self-talk is distracting and consumes energy that is needed to perform the habit or task at hand. Examples of negative self-talk include "I don't like this," "I don't feel like exercising," "I'm tired," and "I can't do this." *Positive* self-talk, on the other hand, has arousal-producing effects and consists of talking to oneself using uplifting, positive statements. Samples include "I can do this," "I feel good," "just three more minutes to go," and "hang in there."

Perfectionism. Perfectionism is a psychological condition, or disposition, in which anything short of perfection is unacceptable. Perfectionists are usually people whose standards are very high, even beyond reach or reason. It is important to eliminate that inner voice or to filter out the voices of others reminding us that "we are still not good enough" or that "something can be better."

Perfectionism has positive and negative forms. Having high standards, positive perfectionism, is fine. Perfectionists are high achievers, persist longer on task, and achieve more than nonperfectionists. Negative perfectionism, however, consists of unreachable and unachievable goals, and the person is almost never satisfied. The perfectionist's expectations of others are also excessive. Positive perfectionists set reasonable goals and recognize when they are achieved. Developing and maintaining healthy habits must be accompanied by patience; making mistakes; and achieving short-term, realistic goals. Negative perfectionism impedes these processes.

Lack of social support. Social support consists of receiving assistance, either directly or indirectly, in physical or mental form, from others (e.g., friends, partners, family, supervisors, mental health professionals) in attempting to reach any goal or to maintain any pursuit. Social support has an important role in learning new habits because it meets many personal needs. Examples of these needs include receiving positive feedback, establishing friendships, and engaging in conversations that encourages the person to "keep going," and it helps alleviate boredom of engaging in a new habit all alone and without company. Sources of social support in exercise settings include exercising with a partner; exercising in a group setting; meeting others at the fitness club who exercise at the same time and establishing friendships; receiving support from family members; working with a personal trainer; or receiving positive feedback from others, which has reinforcement value and promotes feelings of competence and enjoyment.

Perhaps the key issue in determining and reacting to physical and mental barriers—perceived and actual—is one's level of self-control and self-motivation. If a client feels compelled to begin and adhere to a new (healthier) habit and will apply all personal resources (e.g., effort, energy, "must have" outcomes, recruiting social support, a sense of competence in achieving goals, a sense of purpose about linking core values with new rituals), then most if not all perceived barriers—and many actual barriers—can be overcome. Taking control of one's life means not being "a victim" to circumstances, limitations, and others who impede the journey toward a fuller life. Get the negative people out of your way and take control of your destiny. Start telling yourself uplifting, "can-do" stories about your mission—then go after it!

References

Brinthaupt, T. M., Kang, M., & Anshel, M. H. (2010). A delivery model for overcoming psycho-behavioral barriers to exercise. *Psychology of Sport & Exercise, 11*, 259–266.

Buckworth, J., & Dishman, R.K. (1999). Determinants of physical activity: Research to application. *Lifestyle Medicine*, 1016–1027.

Kruger, J., Yore, M.M., Bauer, D.R., & Kohl III, H.W. (2007). Selected barriers and incentives for worksite health promotion services and policies. *American Journal of Health Promotion, 21*, 439–447.

Lox, C.L., Martin, K.A., & Petruzzello, S.J. (2014). *The psychology of exercise: Integrating theory and practice* (4th ed.). Scottsdale, AZ: Holcomb Hathaway.

Markland, D., & Ingledew, D.K. (1997). The measurement of exercise motives: Factorial validity and invariance across gender of a revised Exercise Motivations Inventory. *British Journal of Health Psychology, 2*, 361–376.

Salmon, J., Owen, N., Crawford, D., Bauman, A., & Sallis, J. F. (2003). Physical activity and sedentary behavior: A population-based study of barriers, enjoyment, and preference. *Health Psychology, 22*, 178–188.

Timmerman, G.M. (2007). Addressing barriers to health promotion in underserved women. *Family and Community Health, Supplement, 1*, S34–S42.

PART V

Cognitive and Behavioral Strategies That Promote Healthy Habits

14

DEFINING AND EXPLAINING COGNITIVE AND BEHAVIORAL STRATEGIES

Developing new, healthy habits takes time, effort, and plenty of self-motivation. The primary goal, of course, is to change one's lifestyle to improve health, happiness, energy, and quality of life. While there have been an array of published and marketed programs and interventions to meet this growing need, relatively few of these address specific and effective techniques. These techniques are collectively referred to as *cognitive* (i.e., thoughts/mental skills) and *behavioral strategies* (i.e., actions) that are intended to favorably influence the client's thoughts, emotions, and actions. Because these interventions and strategies have been validated through research and published in a scientific journal, they are usually called "evidence-based."

It would be fair to say that researchers and practitioners differ on what constitutes a "proven" technique. Practitioners give more credit to "hands-on," personal experience that reflects what has worked for them in the past than what researchers tend to offer. It remains clear that the effectiveness of various types of techniques differs from person to person. It is also important that health professionals *not provide too many techniques at one time*. It is easy for clients/patients to become overwhelmed by being asked to learn, think about, and use an array of techniques, or mental skills, too quickly before the mental skill has been learned and performed effectively. New techniques should be introduced one at a time until each has been integrated into one's repertoire of mental skills.

Preliminary Issues for Using Health-Related Strategies

What are some of the reasons people struggle with replacing old (undesirable) habits with new routines that result in better health, more energy, higher life satisfaction (connected to their values), and performance? Here are a few suggestions for overcoming resistance to health behavior change.

Overcoming the perceived lack of time excuse. Having "not enough time" to adopt to new habits, including exercise, dieting, and reducing stress, is a very frequent perception. This is what health professionals need to know to respond to this client excuse.

(1) There are 168 hours in a week (24 hours x 7 days). The exercise science research literature indicates that people should engage in cardiovascular exercise at least three hours a week, preferably on alternative days (e.g., Monday, Wednesday, Friday), to obtain the health- and fitness-related benefits of an exercise habit.
(2) Three hours out of 168 hours in a week equals exercising for only 1.5% of one's week.
(3) Therefore, a person who asserts that the reason for not exercising is "not enough time" is not providing a valid excuse. The real message here is that exercise is not a high priority in the person's daily and weekly "to do" list. So, sure, if you make 99% of your daily activities more important than exercise, it's easy to see why there is insufficient time to exercise or to integrate any other habit into one's daily routine.
(4) According to information provided on the Internet, cell phone use in many countries averages 14–22 hours a week (8–13%, depending on the age group), while watching television can be up to 25–28 hours a week (15–16%). These figures are consistent for people with full-time employment.

The important point here is that many people do not consider new habits, including various forms of exercise, an integral part of their lifestyle. Here are a few of the reasons.

Exercise overtraining. While it is well known that physical training and getting in shape improve health and are imperative in preparation for sports competition, sometimes exercise and other forms of physical activity can be overdone. In fact, there is a body of research literature that reflects a condition called *exercise dependence* or *addiction* that reflects a person's compulsion to exercise regularly in order to feel fulfilled and happy. Addictions are, by definition, undesirable because of the person's inability to control the need, desire, and dependence to engage in the addicted behavior(s).

Exercise burnout. Relatively few former athletes continue to engage in regular exercise after their sport careers end. This may partly be due—or completely due—to the athlete's former sports coach who may have required athletes to exercise excessively or found it necessary to use exercise as a form of punishment. That's called *overtraining.* Exercising an athlete "to death," otherwise called overtraining, can lead to long-term, even permanent, negative attitudes toward physical activity—exercise burnout—after the athlete's retirement from sport.

Studies are apparently absent concerning the degree of postretirement exercise habits among former college athletes. However, interviews with over 300 former college athletes during my academic career clearly indicates that they no longer had any interest in exercising after their college sport careers ended. They explained that overexercising/overtraining during their playing days was the main reason. Sadly, most college athletes gain excessive weight as a result of their post-retirement negative attitude toward exercise and subsequent sedentary lifestyle, despite maintaining their abundant appetites.

Exercise as punishment. Athletes and students in physical education classes may be exercising excessively against their will due to their PE teachers' insistence. Exercise or sports training may be used by many sports coaches as a form of punishment ("You made an error so take 10 laps"). Where did we, as a culture, learn this terrible habit of requiring students and athletes to run laps or perform other forms of exercise as punishment for the student's/athlete's transgression? Is there not a better way to punish or discipline a child for misbehavior? Dr. Monica O'Rourke (2011) found that having a negative experience in high school physical education class contributed to the decision to lead a sedentary lifestyle as middle-aged adults.

Injury. Any form of physical activity may result in injury, and it is wrong to exercise when injured. Tissue damage can become more extensive. You have to "listen" to your body and rest and heal if feeling discomfort due to an injury. In fact, often an overweight or obese person is more susceptible to pain and injury than his or her normal-weight counterpart due to the pressure the obese person places on his or her lower limbs during physical activity. Past studies have shown that fitness, both aerobic and strength related, improves stability around joints and makes us *less* likely to feel physical discomfort. In addition, less body weight reduces the amount of pressure on lower limb joints, thereby preventing injury in the first place.

Lack of fitness knowledge. Exercise is a science. Becoming more fit through a program of regular physical activity and exercise is among the types of physical activity needed to improve fitness and requires expert coaching and applying the exercise science literature. Going for a casual walk will not improve one's fitness, for instance. Leading a sedentary lifestyle all week, then jogging or exercising on the weekend to make up for lost time and training will also fail to lead to reaching desirable fitness goals. Correct exercise technique is a learned set of skills that requires continued practice. Proper instruction on getting started in your fitness program, testing (i.e., pretesting to use as a baseline against which to compare future test scores—the post-test), learning correct methods to lift weights (i.e., resistance training), and discovering ways to gain strength and cardio fitness safely and without injury are necessary to help prevent quitting an exercise program. This rarely happens, however, particularly for novices. New fitness club members, for instance, are often left alone to use the facilities, not knowing proper protocol nor given instruction—unless they pay an additional fee beyond club membership. For many individuals, this added expense is excessive. The fitness club industry can improve its service when it comes to helping participants, especially novice exercisers, improve their fitness levels.

Unpleasant sensations from vigorous physical activity. Exercise does not feel good for everyone. Many individuals find physical exertion to be unpleasant, even unbearable if the person is overweight, unfit, or suffers from a former or current injury. Our threshold of discomfort from physical activity differs. One reason for this is that we are who we train to be. If people lead a sedentary lifestyle and become overweight, their bodies are "trained" to be comfortable with that lifestyle. The body's physiology is not able to adjust to the added stress of increased physical exertion, also called "expanding one's physical capacity" or having "a training effect." Poor exercise technique and inadequate footwear (shoes with poor foot support) make matters worse.

Our sedentary lifestyle. How lazy are we as a culture? How much do we tend to disdain moving our body and become physically active? Try observing the number of people who just stand on an escalator going *down*, rather than walk down the stairs as the escalator is moving. Why do people spend much of their time at home sitting, as opposed to occasional physical activity such as walking, cleaning, or gardening? Many cultures breed inactivity and eating large portions, while others (e.g., the Scandinavian countries of Sweden, Norway, Finland, and Denmark) encourage physical activity as much as possible while eating low-fat foods in small or moderate portions. This is why it is so important to encourage clients to move—to do anything active such as gardening, walking stairs, or riding a bicycle—anything that encourages physical activity on a daily basis. When it comes to structured exercise, it is imperative to start slow then build up resistance to fatigue and discomfort over time.

Strategies that Promote Exercise Performance

It's important to define a cognitive strategy (mental skill), a cognitive-behavioral program, and an intervention.

Defining Terms

Interventions

Starting and maintaining a new habit requires conscious planning of location, time, and behavior. These steps, collectively called an *intervention*, include one or more strategies, subcategorized as cognitive—what a person thinks—or behavioral—a person's actions—that are supposed to change some predetermined outcome (Singer & Anshel, 2006). The primary goal of an intervention is to help individuals adopt to one or more new rituals (e.g., regular exercise, food intake, managing stress). Interventions determine which strategies are needed to build rituals that result in certain specific outcomes.

An *intervention* is a global concept that includes all types of cognitive and behavioral strategies and mental skills that are intended to improve performance outcomes. In sport and physical activity settings, Singer and Anshel (2006) define an intervention as "the process by which sport psychologists attempt to influence the thoughts, emotions, or performance quality of sports competitors and teams" (p. 63). Health professionals, then, are persons who "intervene" by positioning themselves or their strategies between the client and the environment or situation to alter the person's thoughts (e.g., positive self-talk), emotions (e.g., happiness, enthusiasm), and/or actions (e.g., exercise) in a favorable manner. The health professional provides information and instruction to clients about the proper use of one or more mental or behavioral strategies and interventions.

What makes an intervention effective? Researchers have tested the effectiveness of specific cognitive or behavioral strategies and interventions on changes in behavior. Many effective strategies, such as environmental stimuli that prompt certain behavioral responses, called cues-to-action; self-monitoring (i.e., keeping records of progress, including ratings of perceived and activity logs); goal setting; music; personalized performance coaching/personal training; social support; and positive instructional feedback have been shown to improve performance and the development of healthy habits (Anshel, 2014).

Treatments

Despite being used interchangeably in the literature, the terms "treatments" and "interventions" are not the same. A *treatment* is a specific mental or physical procedure that should result in a predictable outcome. An *intervention*, however, consists of a series of treatments or a program that may consist of several types of treatments. A sample treatment might consist of providing instruction on proper diet and nutrition or correct presleep strategies that will help ensure a better night of sleep. A dietary intervention, on the other hand, would require the individual to learn and apply multiple treatments, such as avoiding a full meal at least three hours before bedtime, focusing on activities that decrease arousal level, not watching "high excitement" television, and avoiding cardiovascular exercise within two to three hours before bedtime. Combining exercise with other lifestyle habits that promote health (e.g., nutrition coaching, stress management, other lifestyle changes that improve mental well-being) is an intervention.

Strategies

Strategies are self-initiated mental or physical activities that ostensibly improve some predetermined outcome or goal. If the strategy consists of the person's thoughts, it's called a *cognitive strategy*. A cognitive strategy: (1) improves cognition, that is, the processing of visual, auditory, and tactual input, or (2) favorably influences the client's emotions, such as reducing anxiety, improving attentional focusing, maintaining concentration, and coping with stress (Anshel, 2006).

Strategies are intended to improve performance quality and outcomes. Examples of *cognitive* strategies include positive self-talk, anticipation, precueing and cueing, psyching up, a variety of coping skills, various relaxation techniques, and visualization (also called mental imagery). Sample *behavioral* strategies—discussed later in this book—include recording performance outcomes, developing and using a self-monitoring checklist, exercising with a friend and other forms of social support, receiving instruction or positive feedback, and exercise as therapy. The next chapter consists of explaining some of the more common cognitive strategies related to exercise.

References

Anshel, M. H. (2005). *Applied exercise psychology: A practitioner's guide to client health and fitness*. New York: Springer Publishing Company.

Anshel, M.H. (2014). *Applied health fitness psychology*. Champaign, IL: Human Kinetics.

O'Rourke, M. (2011). *Predictors of attitudes toward physical activity as a function of secondary school physical education experiences among adults*. A doctoral dissertation at Middle Tennessee State University, Murfreesboro, TN.

Singer, R.N., & Anshel, M.H. (2006). An overview of interventions in sport. In J. Dosil (Ed.), *The sport psychologist's handbook* (pp. 64–88). New York: Wiley.

15

COGNITIVE STRATEGIES FOR HEALTH BEHAVIOR CHANGE

How can cognitive strategies—mental skills—encourage the use of healthy habits? Here is a brief review of selected cognitive strategies (sometimes called mental skills) that can answer this question. For more information about cognitive strategies in sport and exercise settings, consult most sport psychology textbooks.

Positive Self-Talk (PST)

Changing habits is easier if accompanied by self-statements that are uplifting, motivating, and confidence-building. Positive self-talk also helps reduce anxiety and other negative moods that impede effort and distract the person from engaging in the new habit with undivided attention. The result will be more effort, better regulation of emotional intensity, heightened concentration, and greater enjoyment of the task.

Another reason to engage in PST is to analyze physical skills and movements that will lead to better performance. For example, PST may be used to anticipate the new habit—let's say dental flossing—rehearse how to perform it, and/or to conduct a postperformance analysis of the habit. "How did the new habit (e.g., going for a rapid walk on your street) feel during and after performing it?" "Did it work, and meet my goal(s)?" "What do I need to do better next time?" A key word in this strategy is "positive." Self-statements, such as "Stay with it," "Concentrate on the task, "I can do this," "Focus," or "I'm feeling better" offer strong motivation, confidence, encouragement, and favorable future expectations to handle the physical demands associated with exercise and other forms of vigorous physical activity. Other examples of self-talk in exercise settings include "Let's do it," "I feel good," and "Stay with it." The uses of single words that influence mood are also effective, such as "Go," "Focus," and "Get it!"

Mental Imagery

Mental imagery, also called *visualization*, is used for several different reasons, such as mentally rehearsing new skills and strategies, detecting and overcoming errors, building self-confidence, developing automated routines, and managing discomfort or pain. After the purpose of a particular imagery session has been determined, clients take a few minutes to relax with eyes closed. Then they generate a mental image that is "performed perfectly" in their mind and always with a successful outcome. Performing the new healthy habit can be visualized and rehearsed before being carried out.

Bizarre Imagery

The purpose of bizarre imagery is to increase performance motivation, both short term and long term. While normal imagery is a mental representation of *actual* performance, bizarre imagery is a mental representation of unrealistic events. For example, cancer patients are sometimes asked to imagine their tumors being shrunk as they receive chemotherapy. Cardiac or pulmonary patients might imagine rapid changes in their circulatory system during an exercise bout that are, otherwise, medically impossible (e.g., enlargement of blood vessels or expansion of lungs). An overweight person might imagine fat being "dissolved". The technique is called "bizarre" because the imagined processes cannot actually occur, and yet these images have strong motivational value.

Thought-stopping

A common dilemma in learning a new habit—even thinking about it—is engaging in unpleasant self-statements about the task or preferred outcome at hand. Unpleasant feelings, especially if continued while performing the new habit, such as having unpleasant thoughts when trying to get to sleep, may lead to reduced motivation and effort or even quitting or not adhering to the new habit. Dropping out of a new program is another example. Therefore, thought-stopping should be used when experiencing negative feelings; clients/patients should say to themselves "STOP!" Ostensibly, the negative thought should diminish; the command to "stop" serves as a verbal cue to replace unpleasant thoughts with more positive ones.

Psyching Up

For some activities, such as the exertion of physical exercise that often requires high arousal and energy, the performer's thought processes must be upbeat and "active." A cognitive strategy called *psyching up* is used to improve task performance that requires high exertion, either briefly or over a brief period of time. The purpose of this strategy is to increase the performer's excitation, sense of challenge, and optimal effort (notice the words "maximal effort" are not used; this is because every task and condition warrants its own unique level of arousal; not every task requires all-out effort).

Psyching up can be experienced in either physical or mental form. Physically, the person can engage in tasks that require increased energy and a higher physiological response, such as higher heart rate, respiration rate, and muscle tension. Mentally, psyching up usually consists of thoughts that increase the performer's confidence, motivation, and arousal while improving attentional focusing and concentration. Examples of psyching-up types of thoughts include "Let's do it," and "I'm ready." Soon after using these "arousal-inducing" terms should come explosive effort to meet performance goals.

Dissociation

The important goal in pain management or recovery from injury is to separate the patients' minds from their bodies. This technique consists of a cognitive strategy called *dissociation*. Dissociation attempts to separate one's attentional focus from physical exertion and, instead, to focus on external stimuli or events. Instead of focusing on the discomfort of pain or fatigue, for example, individuals focus on a predetermined external stimulus, such as music, the fitness instructor, a wall clock, or some other environmental cue not linked to physical exertion. Other examples when dissociation is best used include distance running or someone undergoing physical rehabilitation whose therapy requires movements that are uncomfortable. Dissociation is often used by individuals engaged in endurance or long-term tasks such as jogging, ways to get to sleep, or coping with stress. When clients focus their attention on external stimuli, they are ignoring their own sensations, including pain, physical fatigue, and discomfort.

Association

The conscious attempt at linking the mind and body is called *association*. Sometimes association is used to confront or link thoughts or emotions with behavior. An example of properly using association is during strength training in which the lifter's attentional focus is *internal*, that is, on the muscles executing the lift rather than on some aspect of the situation unrelated to the task. Lifting weights is often a required task in rehabilitation programs. To overpower the feelings of discomfort, exercisers use self-statements such as "Focus on the task at hand," or combine association with imagery in which the person is mentally performing the habit or skill while focusing on sensations of the movement. These feelings are then transferred to the actual performance situation.

Mental Toughness

Mental toughness (MT) is traditionally defined as having the *natural* or *developed* psychological edge that enables the person to deal effectively with external demands. The result is more consistent performance, while the performer remains determined, focused, confident, and in control, particularly under pressure. In addition, mentally tough individuals demonstrate emotional resiliency by bouncing back from physical and mental challenges and physical demands.

Mental toughness is not a personality trait; it is learned, not inherited. During high-pressure situations or external demands, including implanting new healthy habits, MT enables clients to control their emotions in order to buffer against stress and pressure, to feel control over the situation, and to respond favorably to pressure and challenges. Defeat and failure are viewed as opportunities for feedback and improvement. MT also enables athletes to rebound swiftly after experiencing negative events. Rather than being a specific technique, MT consists of an array of mental skills and a "style" of thinking.

Relaxation

Relaxation is the reduction or complete absence of muscular activity in the voluntary muscles. Various forms of relaxation have proven very popular because they help reduce anxiety and stress and improve sleep, which are common problems. There are various types of relaxation strategies, each serving different purposes and meeting individual needs. Examples include *progressive relaxation, autogenic training, biofeedback, imagery, centering*, and *hypnosis*. Though full descriptions of these techniques go beyond the scope of this chapter, each strategy serves similar purposes in reducing muscular tension, lowering arousal level, and improving the person's emotional status.

It is important to note, however, that relaxation is not always appropriate and effective in response to stress. Some individuals find they are not compatible with relaxation techniques. They prefer a more active approach to stress reduction such as low-intensity exercise or merely want to be distracted from life's storms. Sample activities for this purpose include watching television or films or socially interacting with others. In addition, some situations do not warrant relaxation outcomes; at times, increased emotional arousal or heightened concentration is warranted. If used correctly, however, relaxation training is a valid and proven means of preventing or reducing muscular tension and anxiety, while improving concentration and self-confidence.

Cognitive strategies are learned (mental) skills. Like any skill, they require instruction, practice, opportunities for learning, feedback, time to master, and individualized consultation so that the client's/patients unique needs are taken into account during consultations. Therapists and coaches should avoid overprescribing these techniques. Allow client's/patients to apply and learn each technique under simulated-then-actual conditions.

16

BEHAVIORAL STRATEGIES FOR HEALTH BEHAVIOR CHANGE

A *behavioral* strategy, as opposed to a cognitive strategy, consists of one or more conscious (usually observable) *actions* that are intended to improve a predetermined performance quality or outcome. Sample behavioral strategies include exercising in rhythm to (or background) music; light exercise to reduce stress or anxiety; goal setting (example of a nonobservable behavioral strategy); and social support such as exercising with a partner, self-monitoring, scheduling, and record keeping.

Behavioral strategies are always intentional and purposeful, not coincidental, subconscious, or unintended. Both cognitive and behavioral strategies are used to improve or regulate the person's emotions, increase the speed or efficiency of information processing (e.g., having positive self-expectations, anticipating a stimulus, storing and retrieving information from memory, increasing speed of decision-making), and achieving a goal such as optimal performance. Sample behavioral strategies follow.

Physical Location

Previous studies have shown that adherence to new habits is far more likely if the person does not have to travel more than three miles out of the way between home and work. It is important, therefore, that clients need not travel too far outside their normal commute or from home or work to use an exercise facility or visit a specialist who will help them initiate a new routine or behavior pattern. It is increasingly likely clients will adhere to a new ritual if they perceive the environment in which they intend to execute the new behavior as safe.

What about initiating the new habit at home? Using a home-based exercise program as an example, there is a reason that home exercise equipment often goes unused (except to hang clothes to dry). We tend to associate our home with relaxation, recreation, entertainment, and recovery from life's storms. We do not link home with hard physical exertion, perspiration, and working out. It is not surprising, therefore, that many individuals tend to purchase exercise equipment with the best of intentions (especially following New Year's resolutions and gifts from others) then stop using it—or never start. For some individuals, exercise is best performed in the company of others, perhaps in an atmosphere that increases a person's arousal level and provides incentive and energy to go all-out, such as an exercise facility or a group exercise class rather than the solitude of exercising alone.

Scheduling

Routines and new/healthy habits that are scheduled bring some degree of order and structure to our life, which needs structure to be productive and achieve our goals. Attempts to replace a person's current, unhealthy habits with new, more desirable ones is enormously difficult, partly because change is—for many people—uncomfortable and "risky." The chance of developing a new habit, however, is far more likely if the new thought, emotion, or behavior is planned and scheduled in advance. *Plans that are more detailed are more likely to be carried out.* Clients, in conjunction with their health professional or coach, should select days of the week and the "best," most convenient time of day that is most likely to result in carrying out and adhering to the new habit.

One word of caution to health professionals. Scheduling a new habit is more effective if it is convenient to the client's current schedule and location, particularly in the presence of a social support agent such as a coach, instructor, or mental health professional. The new habit should be as consistent and undisruptive as possible to the person's current habits and lifestyle. For example, it is well known in the scientific community that certain behaviors should be avoided within two to three hours before bedtime. These include eating a full meal, engaging in cardiovascular exercise, and any experience or thought that induces high stress. According to the National Sleep Foundation (www.nationalsleepfoundation.org), televisions should not be located in the bedroom (which 70% of U.S. homes do have). The reason is that most TV content, especially in the evenings, increases arousal (i.e., heart rate, respiration rate, negative emotions, even aggression level) and impedes rather than promotes sleep. See the NSF website to obtain presleep rituals at www.sleepfoundation.org/publications.

Individualized Coaching

For many individuals, a behavioral strategy begins with receiving personal attention and instruction as well as feeling accountable to someone of perceived importance (e.g., a coach, mental health professional, medical practitioner). Many people need this form of social support when embarking on a journey to improve their health, happiness, and energy. Starting a new routine can be stressful. Fear of failure, noncompliance, and lack of knowledge about the way to properly carry out the new ritual cause anxiety and failure to meet performance goals. For novice exercisers, for instance, some of the many unknowns are: (a) Will I be able to exercise without pain? (b) Will I hurt myself when being physically active? (c) I have not exercised since I was a kid; I don't know what to do or how to do it. (d) Will I look awkward to others who see me? (e) Will others, who are fitter, thinner, and/or younger, mock or laugh at me? (f) Will I have time to continue my exercise program? (g) I hated exercising in high school; why am I doing this now? Novices bring with them thoughts of previous exercise attempts, fears about experiencing injury or fatigue, and how the body will respond to new physical demands to a new program. Heightened self-consciousness about one's appearance, doubts about meeting performance goals, and not being taught the correct way to exercise only worsen these initial feelings of doubt and pessimism.

Any novice exerciser who visits a fitness program or facility needs to be welcomed, comforted (i.e., made to feel accepted and whose needs are important), and informed. The program should include a set of preset routines that help new participants to feel comfortable upon entering the facility, secure a set of pre-exercise routines (e.g., locker room use, availability of services, towels, exercise programs), and make participants feel comfortable starting a particular program. Instruction on proper exercise technique should always be offered at the start of someone's participation, or the participant might experience pain or a debilitating injury.

Someone on staff, particularly a fitness (or membership) coach, should address their members' concerns and how the staff might help them experience a proper and effective exercise session. Established programs should include teaching proper exercise techniques; helping members set realistic goals; and helping them feel secure in an environment filled with uncertainties, intimidation, and physical and emotional challenges. Novice exercisers need to feel they are "fitting in," accepted, respected, and not self-conscious about their lack of prior training and current physical appearance. The failure to personally and professionally connect with clients will almost certainly lead to dropping out of the program, or at least not renewing their membership.

Psychological Services/Mental Skills Coaching

A number of questions and issues needs to be addressed on this topic. Dropping out of programs often has deep roots in one's past and might be alleviated with counseling. What is the purpose of offering mental health professional (MHP) services to program participants/patients? If this is a counseling service, then a person who is credentialed to render therapy is required. If, however, this service is about goal setting and performance enhancement strategies, then a different service is being offered, similar to what athletes experience with sport psychologists. Should a person attending a fitness club or physical rehabilitation program have access to an MHP through the program he or she is attending? Or should this type of service be separate from the program? What would be the MHP's role and responsibility if located within the fitness or rehabilitation program area? What issues would be addressed? Would it be performance based or include psychotherapy? How could the client be assured that all information would be strictly confidential?

Several other issues need to be addressed. For instance, where would the service be offered, at the exercise venue (likely in a private room/office) or in another facility where the MHP has an office? How can fitness club management and MHPs make this service available to *all* club exercisers, not just novices and not only those who seek it? This service must be kept confidential and unknown to anyone other than the client. Who would pay for this service? Insurance? The client? How would this service be promoted, and what issues would be addressed?

Would the MHP work in coordination with personal trainers in trying to help the client improve fitness, prevent dropping out, and learn to use proper performance-enhancing strategies? While it is clear clinical services are sometimes needed to address an individual's psychological needs in order to feel more comfortable in an exercise program, less certain is where and how this service should be provided. What would be the MHPs title? Performance Consultant/Counselor? Psychologist? Mental Health Coach?

This service can focus on the following issues, some of which would include building new habits: (a) performance-related issues such as improving motivation and mental toughness, (b) building confidence, (c) managing anxiety related to exercise participation, (d) teaching clients how to use exercise as a means of stress reduction, (e) helping clients set and achieve challenging goals, (f) teaching the proper use of mental skills that enhance exercise performance (psyching up, imagery, and others discussed later), (g) providing social support by perhaps matching a client with someone else with similar characteristics, (h) linking the strengths of each personal trainer with the unique needs of each client, (i) addressing eating disorders and other obstacles to proper dieting and problem eating, and (j) acting as the liaison for participants who need to communicate with club staff or someone to whom they can turn for advice. Some of these issues require a state-recognized credential such as certification or licensure. Currently there are apparently no studies examining the effectiveness and usefulness of a mental skills coach program.

Goal Setting

Setting goals is a significant motivator for improving performance, particularly with respect to developing new habits and a healthier lifestyle. The effect of setting goals is *minimal* if a person does not set them correctly; there is little motivational effect. Typically, goals are effective when they are set correctly, and it begins by having the performer play a role in the goal-setting process. Goals must reflect realistic expectations about performance outcomes. It makes no sense for an athlete's coach or an exerciser's personal trainer to set extraordinarily difficult goals that, the client feels, are unattainable. The result of setting excessive goals is demotivation.

Goals should include both short-term and long-term objectives, focus on performance quality (not only outcomes), be moderately challenging to improve confidence and task adherence, and be quantifiable (numerical). There should be a clear indication if the goal was met. Poorly set goals can promote feelings of helplessness and lead to dropping out of the program.

Sample goals in exercise settings include: "I will complete 20 minutes nonstop on the treadmill at a speed of *x* miles per hour at an elevation of 1"; "I will complete three sets of eight repetitions each when lifting 40 pounds"; or "I will reach my training heart rate during five work-rest interval training sessions, each of which consists of running for three minutes then walking for 30 seconds." Notice that these goals are *performance* (process) goals, rather than *outcome* (product) goals (e.g., "I will lose three pounds" or "I will decrease 2% body fat"), which are long-term, not short-term, goals and not under the exerciser's self-control. In nonexercise settings that promote healthy habits, sample goals are: "I will wear my CPAP mask (to overcome sleep apnea) for the full night and not remove it before I wake up in the morning, restroom needs notwithstanding"; "I will follow my diet for the next seven days"; "I will avoid eating dinner within two hours of bedtime"; "I will go walking after dinner each night"; and "I will give my spouse a hug (kiss) each day before I leave for work."

Social Support

The role of social support in building positive, healthy habits has been discussed earlier. Nevertheless, the role of others in promoting health behavior change has been well established in the literature. While some people prefer to be left alone and to learn a new habit alone, many others prefer to feel supported by others during the process of learning new behaviors, especially when these actions are life changing. The process of being assisted and helped by others is called *social support.*

The need for social support is especially important when the individual lacks confidence, is uncertain about his or her ability to succeed at the new habit, or the person welcomes the companionship of others for motivation purposes. Companionship can be a strong motivator to meet performance goals and challenges, especially for the novice exerciser. Some individuals prefer the company of others, especially if they feel self-conscious about their physical appearance or they find that being accountable to another person—perhaps their coach—provides the incentive to adhere to their program.

Nonverbal/secondary/indirect forms of social support consist of ways to facilitate the exerciser's ability to develop and maintain the new habit, such as providing transportation, giving a fitness club membership or diet program as a gift, encouraging the person to maintain their new habit, and supervising or monitoring the person's progress. As Sarafino (1994) contends "people are more likely to start and stick with (a new habit such as exercise) if these efforts have the support and encouragement of family and friends" (p. 267).

Rewards

According to positive social reinforcement theory, rewards have information value about a person's perception of competence. A reward, such as a t-shirt, certificate, or a gift, recognizes the person's achievement and enhances his or her sense of accomplishment and group member identification. Both outcomes markedly improve participation satisfaction and adherence to new routines and healthy habits. In order to build intrinsic motivation, that is, feelings of satisfaction, enjoyment, and competence, it is best to link the reward directly to a desirable performance outcome or achievement, such as jogging a specific, predetermined distance or adhering to a particular diet, rather than as a response to participation that the person expects.

Educational Materials

The written word is a powerful tool in helping people to understand the value of what they can do to improve their health. While it is best to avoid exposing clients to complicated, difficult to understand research journal articles in providing information, other sources might be more understandable, such as magazine or newspaper articles, segments of books, and even materials created by the health professional. These "homemade" materials provide clients with a better understanding and justification for their habits and the techniques needed to learn and maintain them. Monthly newsletters with featured articles that address ways to learn and adhere to different types of healthy habits and findings from recent studies all have great motivational value.

Memberships in Clubs, Organizations, and Programs

A behavioral strategy that helps meet the personal and social needs of most people related to health behavior is to join a club or organization—or to be part of a structured program, either in person or through a website. Running or bicycling clubs, groups who meet for weekly lectures or other functions, banquets that recognize fitness achievement, exercise-related events (e.g., weekend jogging or biking), company or individual-sponsored contests (e.g., "The John Smith Annual Run"), outdoor activity clubs, annual guest speaker or award events, health-related conferences or seminars (especially popular with weight loss clubs and programs), and exhibitions (e.g., power lifting, aerobic dance) are sample behavioral strategies—activities—that create excitement and motivation to start and maintain a new healthy habit.

Environmental Features

Another behavioral strategy concerns arranging the exercise environment to provide clients with greater excitement and incentive for making the journey toward improving health by adopting one or more new habits. These incentives can include colorful walls; equipment that is properly working, modern, and clean; and any other conditions that provide a pleasant and professional atmosphere. Broken equipment should be fixed as soon as possible, particularly if the participant relies on this equipment to adhere to the new habit. Water fountains are notoriously out of order and need to be fixed immediately to provide clients with hydration. Broken equipment communicates a sense of insensitivity ("We want your membership money but do not care about providing a valuable service that you want") and poor management ("We are not in touch with program needs") and reduces credibility of the service being provided by not taking the necessary steps to provide high-quality and professional environment. Facilities in which new habits are adopted (e.g., exercise, massage, manicure/pedicure) need to appear ready to use and be of high quality.

In addition, important information about any facility in which the new habit will be formed should be easily accessible at the front counter, such as reprints on articles and other educational materials, business cards of staff, scheduled special programs, sales, and general information (e.g., hours of operation, membership costs, who to see if a particular question or issue needs to be addressed).

Finally, the facility should include staff who are friendly and well informed so they can answer client questions, be genuine about helping others, be professionally dressed, and express a sincere and trusting demeanor toward clients. For example, licensed psychologists are affiliated with most departments of law enforcement. They may provide counseling to selected department personnel related to experiencing a traumatic event, managing stress, dealing with both personal and work-related issues, and acting as a liaison between them and the department administration. Users of this service must, first, trust the MHP so that all interaction content will be kept strictly confidential. It must be understood that issues addressed in therapeutic sessions will not be shared with others.

Record Keeping

It is normal to feel motivated in response to improvement and competence, an issue that is at the heart of intrinsic motivation (IM). Briefly, IM is a type of motivation that reflects a person's decision to perform a skill or engage in a task for the sake of pleasure, enjoyment, or a sense of achievement. One objective measure to detect improvement and achievement, which increases IM, is through testing and obtaining quantitative data.

Health professionals might consider recording baseline measures that are changeable over a reasonable time period (usually within three to four months) then monitor the client's progress by maintaining records and retesting (post-testing). Performance data should be recorded, updated, and monitored in quantitative form, reflecting numbers rather than general comments such as "Nancy did a good job today" or "John is feeling better about his exercise progress." The perception of improvement as shown by test scores improves a sense of accomplishment, competence, and satisfaction, all very relevant to IM. It confirms to clients that making optimal effort to achieve goals can be successful and enjoyable. "Seeing on paper how far they have progressed can be very reinforcing," Sarafino (1994, p. 267) contends.

Self-Monitoring Checklist

The behavioral technique associated with developing and maintaining a list of "things to do" is called *self-monitoring*. The checklist consists of listing the thoughts, emotions, and actions that should be part of the person's protocol to learn and maintain new habits. Checklists are not "tests" because tests infer "right" and "wrong" answers. Rather, checklists provide a set of guidelines about properly learning and executing the new habit under pleasant, correct, and efficient conditions. Thus, a score of "5" for each checklist item is always desirable. Items that are scored 1, 2, or 3 require the client's and the health professional's attention in attempting to raise that score. *The goal in completing this checklist is to improve the total score for each component.*

For the novice exerciser, for instance, fitness coaches should review the checklist at least once per week but usually *less* often after the first month of use. Eventually, perhaps after several weeks of regular monitoring, the checklist will serve as an occasional reminder of pre-exercise and exercise rituals. With time, these rituals (e.g., drinking water within 10 minutes of the exercise session; warming up by walking before jogging) will become habits. Therefore, maintaining the checklist is more important at earlier stages of developing exercise routines, while a checklist eventually becomes less important with time and experience.

An additional issue is that selected items on the checklist may be irrelevant to some individuals. For example, some individuals would rather exercise alone rather than exercising with others, which runs counter to the item about "exercises with others." Both conditions, exercise alone or with others, are normal. Therefore, the item that addresses exercising in a group setting versus exercising alone can be eliminated from the checklist if the exerciser actually prefers to be alone when working out. Other items that are contrary to the exerciser's needs and preferences can also be eliminated, as long as omitting the item will not induce quitting or injury. A separate inventory has been developed for persons who may be addicted to exercise: Exercise Dependence Scale—Revised (Symons Downs, Hausenblaus, & Nigg, 2004). Appendix B provides a sample self-monitoring checkist for exercise and improved fitness.

Provide Regular Performance Feedback

Feedback following physical performance skills is inherent to learning and improving. When we follow a certain dietary regimen or use particular relaxation techniques, we anticipate desirable outcomes. When these outcomes are disappointing, we need to determine the reasons, which requires feedback. What procedures were followed correctly and incorrectly? How can we perform a new habit more efficiently and establish a better outcome? Why am I not losing weight after six weeks of my exercise program?

General performance feedback is also a motivational strategy. Health professionals need to acknowledge the client's improved performance, which then increases the client's perceived competence, confidence, and intrinsic motivation. Short-term and long-term adherence often occur if the client finds feedback meaningful, honest, observable, and measurable (e.g., "That was a great effort at completing those repetitions"), rather than reflect more abstract content (e.g., "You're looking better" or "Nice going."). In addition, giving feedback *intermittently* (i.e., regularly; let's say after every few trials) is more effective than giving it *constantly* (i.e., all the time). The important issue here is that clients need to hear and observe positive messages about their performance or about outcomes derived from their efforts if these messages are delivered properly.

Monitor Client Attendance

It may be useful and motivating to keep a record of the client's attendance—perhaps both arrival and departure times if he or she attends a program or facility regularly. These data help determine adherence to the new habit and acknowledge any pattern of absenteeism that might indicate dropping out. Attendance records also might help explain the causes of fitness test results. Absences provide the first warning sign of demotivation and, eventually, quitting the program. One value of recording attendance, if, in fact, attendance reflects the client's commitment to adopt a new (healthy) habit, is to judge the quality of the treatment or intervention. That is, attendance rates help explain the treatment's efficacy and whether a disappointing outcome from the habit can be at least partially explained by noncompliance—not completing the treatment as requested.

Contacting an absent client also communicates a sense of caring and professionalism that clients will appreciate. "Good" attendance after a segment of time (e.g., during *x* number of months) might warrant some form of recognition or some other form of acknowledgement. Self-reported attendance is the primary measure of exercise adherence in the research literature. This can easily occur by having the client sign an attendance sheet after each visit.

Use Small, Attainable Units to Reflect Progress

A person requires information that reflects feelings of achievement on a particular task or toward meeting a specific goal. The result is improving intrinsic motivation. One way to enhance IM is to provide the client with information that reflects improvement and competence in performing the new habit. Usually, there are a series of experiences and information installments that create the client's perceptions of competence over time; the person should be able to detect these increments of improvement, however small. Clients should be provided with small, attainable units that reinforce the clients' perception of moving toward achieving outcome goals. This is why using the relatively small unit of time (minutes, for example, instead of miles) is more likely to reflect competent performance than measuring performance by relatively larger units (e.g., distance/miles).

Perceived Choice

One reason people drop out of exercise classes is because they do not enjoy the type of exercise they are being asked or required to do. To use a cliché, one size does not fit all. It is true that aerobic-type exercise is needed to improve cardiovascular fitness and burn more calories than strength or flexibility exercises. It is inefficient, therefore, to engage in just one type of physical training (e.g., resistance training only) while ignoring others (e.g., aerobic, flexibility). The behavioral strategy of *perceived choice* allows clients to have options about ways to acquire the new habit.

There are, for instance, three different types of CPAP machines for overcoming sleep apnea. All are effective, but only the user can determine their preferred option. Selecting one's own option encourages self-motivation and adherence to the new habit. Clients may find one fitness club more desirable in which to exercise than other clubs. Perceived choice is about providing clients with alternatives that are compatible with their needs. To gain cardiovascular fitness can be accomplished by jogging/running, treadmill, bicycle ergometer, swimming, or some form of physical activity that raises the heart rate and appeals to the exerciser.

Social Engineering

Social engineering is a stress management technique in which persons consciously place themselves in situations or under conditions that reduce or prevent stress. Examples include driving down a less-traveled road and attending an event early before traffic becomes heavy or the venue becomes crowded. A client can avoid a crowded exercise facility by choosing a time to exercise that experiences lower attendance. In addition, it is highly likely the exercise equipment will be more readily available during these "off" hours, and staff will be more available to provide instruction. In addition, for the self-conscious person, lower attendance means less likelihood of being observed by others which can be intimidating.

Music

It is well known, according to scientific studies (e.g., Anshel & Marisi, 1978) and reviews of literature (Karageorghis & Priest, 2010; Karageorghis & Terry, 1997), that music affects physical performance, perhaps, it is thought, by increasing a person's arousal level and improving exercise endurance. One explanation of the benefits of music on physical performance includes the *dissociation effect* in which the performer's attention is focused on external stimuli—the music. At the same time, bodily responses to physical exertion are ignored—or at least receive far less attention.

Another explanation of the benefits of music while exercising is that it increases arousal level due to increased adrenalin flow, which, in turn, ignites the individual's exertion level and effort. The effect is especially beneficial for tasks that requires faster reactions and movement speed. Slower, more relaxing music will, ostensibly, prove more beneficial for less intense sports such as golf, archery, bowling, or slower-moving exercises. It is not surprising that music is almost always playing in exercise facilities; it provides an upbeat mood and motivation to maintain optimal effort.

Modeling

Sometimes exercisers feel intimidated by younger, highly fit, perhaps thinner exercisers, leading to feeling uncomfortable in a public facility where new habits can take hold. One way around feelings of intimidation and anxiety is for the exerciser to observe the performance of a person who has mastered the new habit—if this is feasible, of course. An advanced exerciser and someone involved in stress-reducing activities are examples. This is an especially effective strategy if the client is trying to learn a motor skill in which observing a skilled individual—called the modeling effect—is an effective way to learn.

Time of Day

A very common question asked of exercise novices is "When is the best time of day to exercise?" People differ on the time of day they prefer to exercise, similar to individual differences on preferred bedtime. Some individuals enjoy working out first thing in the morning, while others wake up and the first thing on their mind is getting that first cup of coffee—fast!! Yet others enjoy exercising later in the day, perhaps at lunch time or in the evenings. Some habits should be performed at specific times (e.g., presleep rituals), while other habits can be completed at any time the person feels comfortable and is compatible with his or her schedule.

Time preference for exercise concerns convenience (e.g., "I have more time to exercise after work"; "I prefer to get my workout out of the way so I exercise before work"), body chemistry, and even personality. Studies on time of day for exercise, according to O'Connor and Davis (1992), who confirmed the findings of several earlier Swedish studies, indicate that when we choose to exercise during the day or night does not influence receiving exercise benefits. Early morning exercise routines produce the same benefits as exercising at night. There is one exception to that rule, however.

Researchers have found that it is best *not* to engage in aerobic exercise, or any other type of extreme exertion and stress, within three hours of going to sleep. Researchers have found that sleep is most sound when bedtime is accompanied by a relatively reduced body temperature (i.e., lower heart rate) and low arousal level. Studies also indicate that high-intensity aerobic exercise close to bedtime will reduce time spent in deep sleep. High aerobically fit individuals, however, recover from aerobic exercise faster than their less fit counterparts and, therefore, are not as affected by late night exercise than less fit persons. Therefore, the rule about exercising close to bedtime is more relevant for the person with a low to moderate aerobic fitness level. The bottom line is this: *A person should exercise at a time of day that is convenient and compatible with his or her adherence to a lifestyle that incorporates regular exercise or any other healthy habit.* It is better to exercise or implement any other healthy habit when the person has the opportunity, rather than conforming to some predetermined rule or guideline.

Lifestyle Management

The benefits of improving one's habits, such as changes in dietary habits, improving sleep, reducing stress, and exercise (or some other form of physical activity), do not happen in a vacuum. To obtain optimal benefits, new healthy habits should be incorporated into one's lifestyle that influence a person's energy, work productivity, general physical and mental health, and quality of life. Lifestyle management includes exercise, nutrition, proper rest and sleep, and other rituals that improve physical and mental health and general well-being. The DVM is all about scheduling new rituals that are linked to the client's values in making lifestyle changes, not just a single change in a habit. Self-awareness is about knowing what we have to do to succeed in reaching our destination.

Pedometers

A pedometer is a very inexpensive motion sensor that assesses physical activity, specifically, the number of steps taken per day. It has been used as a device to encourage physical activity. According to Kang et al. (2009) in their extensive review of the pedometer exercise literature, "taking 10,000 steps/day appears to be a reasonable goal of daily activity for healthy adults. Individuals who accumulate 10,000 steps/day are more likely to meet the physical activity guidelines by engaging in the amount of activity promoted by the Centers for Disease Control and Prevention (and other government agencies)" (p. 648). The authors concluded that "the use of pedometers has a moderate and positive effect on the increase of physical activity in intervention studies" (p. 652). Perhaps exercise interventions should include mechanical devices such as pedometers, accelerometers (which includes speed of movement in addition to the number of steps), and a heart rate monitor that measures "target heart rate," that is, exercise intensity to achieve cardiovascular fitness. Each of these devices provides data and information that promote a sense of achievement and improvement.

References

Anshel, M. H., & Marisi, D. Q. (1978). Effect of music and rhythm on physical performance. *Research Quarterly, 49*, 109–113.

Kang, M., Marshall, S.J., Barreira, T.V., & Lee, J. (2009). Effect of pedometer-based physical activity interventions: A meta-analysis. *Research Quarterly for Exercise and Sport, 80*, 648–655.

Karageorghis, C.I., & Priest, D.L. (2010). Music in sport and exercise. An update on research and application. *The Sport Journal, 13*, Internet article. http://thesport journal.org/article/music-sport-and-exercise-update-research-and-application.

Karageorghis, C.I., & Terry, P.C. (1997). The psychophysical effects of music in sport and exercise: A review. *Journal of Sport Behavior, 20*, 54–68.

O'Connor, P.J., & Davis, J.C. (1992). Psychobilogic responses to exercise at different times of day. *Medicine and Science in Sports and Exercise, 24*, 714–719.

Sarafino, E.P. (1994). *Health psychology: Biopsychosocial interactions* (2nd ed.). New York: John C. Wiley & Sons.

Symons Downs, D., Hausenblaus, H.A., & Nigg, C.A. (2004). Factor validity and psychometric examination of the Exercise Dependence Scale—Revised. *Measurement in Physical Education and Exercise Science, 8*, 183–201.

PART VI

Personal Factors That Influence Health Behavior Change

17

PERSONAL QUALITIES THAT *PROMOTE* HEALTHY HABITS

Health deteriorates when people are unhappy, depressed, or stressed, as well as when anxiety consumes their thoughts and actions. Particularly damaging is the lack of self-control—when people feel their life is spiraling out of control, called *helplessness*, and when there is no perception of a better future, called *hopelessness*. These individuals often succumb, even die, due to their tribulations and life's storms. Others, however, are able to overcome strife and focus on what is important to their lives and happiness. They remain optimistic about their future, possess the energy needed to move forward, and maintain healthy habits. This chapter is about describing characteristics of people who deal constructively with life's challenges and storms, who do not allow "bumps in the road" to dictate their happiness, who are relatively tenacious and resistant to stress and pressure, and who feel in control of their destiny.

What Is a Personal Quality?

For the purposes of this chapter and for optimal use of the Disconnected Values Model, *personal qualities* are dispositions and behavioral tendencies that form patterns of thinking and acting that describe and often predict a person's unique characteristics. Researchers have found that certain dispositions are consistent with the self-motivation necessary to adopt healthy habits and to maintain good health. Other dispositions, however, reflect individuals whose habits are not consistent with good health and well-being. The focus of this section is to list and describe the features of a person's thoughts and behaviors—their personal dispositions—that promote a healthy lifestyle.

Confidence: This characteristic is strongly associated with optimistic thinking about the effort needed to reach desirable goals and to anticipate success.

Confident people have more reason to celebrate good health and to ensure that they maintain healthy habits because they are focused on success—current and future—and happiness. Life has meaning; it's purposeful.

Self-esteem: To what extent does a person value himself or herself? What is his or her purpose—his or her value—in life, and how is he or she living a life consistent with that purpose? Self-esteem has multiple components, each independent from each other. Examples include general knowledge (academic), social, sport, and religious, among others. Thus, a person can have high self-esteem in one area—let's say has good social skills—but low self-esteem in other areas; perhaps someone with poor sports skills or exhibits inferior academic performance. People who possess at least one area of high self-esteem are more likely to feel good about themselves and see greater value in maintaining healthy habits than their low self-esteem counterparts.

Self-control (SC): This disposition consists of a set of behaviors that describes a person's self-regulation of emotions and thoughts that, if not controlled, might interfere with high-quality ongoing behavior. This is essential to developing a routine, or habit. SC also helps guide the person through the process of change. People who excel at SC are healthier because they have great command of their thoughts, emotions, and actions, and have the willingness and ability to carry out these processes to their benefit, including improved health. There is no self-destructive behavior pattern for persons with high SC.

Intrinsic motivation (IM): There are several types and definitions of motivation. IM is probably the most desirable and important type of motivation because it reflects a person's self-determination to perform an activity due to his or her high level of satisfaction and perceived competence (PC). Desirable behavior is far more likely to continue when the cause and initiation of that behavior are personal satisfaction, enjoyment, feelings of competence, and fun. High satisfaction and PC result in task persistence—a long-term commitment to engage in a task (see Hagger & Chatzisarantis, 2007 and Roberts & Treasure, 2012 for complete reviews and explanations of intrinsic motivation). Therefore, people who have high IM related to healthy habits are more likely to have positive feelings about and persist in maintaining those habits. High IM reflects a person's tendency to actively develop proper habits, meet challenges, and have an interest in new activities, even without external prompts or rewards. IM is related to self-determination.

Self-determination (SD): SD is a motivational construct. Experiences of competence and autonomy and environmental conditions that support the person's sense of competence and autonomy increase motivation and promote IM, in particular. IM is most likely to take root when the need for relatedness is supported, that is, where people feel a sense of connectedness and belonging to each other and to the group and to meeting individual and group goals. SD is stronger, on the other hand, when people feel relatedness. Feeling rejected and unloved/disrespected, on the other hand, tends to undermine SD and IM. Thus, persons who possess a high degree of SD are more likely to feel responsible and motivated for developing and maintaining healthy habits because they know that good health is linked to desirable outcomes—both for the individual and the group.

Attributional style (AS):AS is a motivational construct consisting of an individual's tendency and preference for how he or she explains both successful and unsuccessful performance outcomes. For instance, a person who explains high-quality performance due to his or her ability will be more motivated to persist at that activity and to retain motivation and confidence in future attempts. Attributing failure to low ability, however, may result in negative emotion, low confidence, and even dropping out of the activity due to feelings of low perceived competence.

Rosenbaum (1990) contends that "Individual differences in attributional style are hypothesized to predict vulnerability to helplessness and depression" (p. xxvi). It is desirable, therefore, that people maintain two internal attribution styles—high ability and high effort—to explain their success, while *not* attributing low ability or low effort following perceived failure. People with an "internal" disposition are more responsible for their actions and, therefore, link their actions to better health.

Hardiness: This concept refers to beliefs that people can adapt to a stressful environment in a healthy manner. They are more capable of meeting challenges and are driven by a commitment to successful outcomes. From his review of this literature, Rosenbaum (1990) concluded that "hardy persons are healthier, less depressed, and perform better than do non-hardy people" (p. xxix).

Rituals: Successful performers believe in structure and preparation, not unlike remembering the importance of practicing healthy habits. Maintaining rituals requires far less physical and mental energy than acting in ways that are unplanned and unpredictable. All high-quality performers have a schedule of their daily routines and can automate most of these actions because they have been well learned.

Competitiveness: Researchers have examined the extent to which successful performers are motivated to win and compete, focus on setting and meeting personal goals, and feel motivated when they win under competitive conditions (which, of course, also carries some risk for losing or failing). Results of these studies show that highly skilled athletes enjoy and optimally strive for success under competitive conditions and tend to measure their success by meeting goals based on performing at or beyond their personal previous best. Competitiveness represents performing at one's best and feeling highly motivated when challenging goals are met. High-quality performers feel their competitive drive from intraindividual comparisons (i.e., comparing their performance with their personal best) rather than interindividual comparisons (i.e., beating the opponent or against a competitor). While the concept of competitiveness has apparently not been studied with respect to maintaining healthy habits, it is reasonable to surmise that competitive individuals have more to lose if they do not properly train and maintain good health. Competitive individuals engage in self-regulation strategies so that they remain in control of their preparation for performance quality.

Learned resourcefulness (LR): Rosenbaum (1990) defines LR as an acquired repertoire of behavioral and cognitive skills with which the person is able to regulate internal events such as emotions and cognitions that might otherwise interfere with the smooth execution of a target behavior (p. xiv). What this means is that healthy individuals possess characteristics that provide the energy and motivation to meet goals and needs by successfully and properly regulating their thoughts, emotions, and actions. They are better than their nonresourceful counterparts in tolerating pain, succeeding in weight reduction/management programs, effective use of coping with stress, and maintaining healthy habits and treatments that will prolong their quality of life and general health.

Mental toughness (MT): Jones, Hanton, and Connaughton (2007) define MT as a psychological disposition that enables a person to cope effectively with life's demands. Mentally tough people are better and more consistent in remaining determined, concentrated, confident, and in control of situations while under pressure. Clough, Earle, and Sewell (2002) view mental toughness as consisting of "individuals [who] tend to be sociable and outgoing as they are able to remain calm and relaxed, they are competitive in many situations and have lower anxiety levels than others" (p. 38). Thus, mentally tough individuals are able to overcome life's obstacles, are unwavering in controlling their future, and have the ability to remain largely unaffected by adverse situations. Maintaining good health is central to having the energy to stay focused on meeting goals, overcoming adverse conditions, and remaining in control of one's destiny.

Need for Achievement (Nach): People who are driven to stay focused on performance goals and have a strong need to succeed, especially in achievement conditions (e.g., competition, being evaluated by others, attempts to meet personal goals) possess a personality trait called *need achievement*. People who have high scores on this trait are called need achievers; they are attracted to achievement conditions, that is, situations in which competence and success are identified. In addition, high need achievers feel greater motivation when they succeed under achievement conditions, such as completing a task or experiencing success under competitive conditions. Good health and maintaining healthy habits are central to achievement.

Expectations for success: Also called the self-fulfilling prophecy, expectations for success is represented by optimism, confidence, and challenging but reasonable goals. The basic premise of this thought process is that we are more likely to be successful and to meet our expectations if we anticipate success. Healthier people maintain expectations for success and life satisfaction because they link healthy habits with desirable performance outcomes. It's as if high expectations are followed by behaviors that are consistent with those expectations. It might follow this line of thinking: "If I exercise vigorously on a regular basis, I will more likely maintain a proper body weight, have more energy, and feel better both mentally and physically than if I sit all day and do not exercise." If we expect success, we tend to conduct ourselves in ways that promote success. Researchers call it the *expectancy effect*.

In summary, while researchers cannot claim that having certain personality traits or dispositions can accurately predict good—or bad—health, the results of numerous studies suggest that certain dispositions are strongly related to good health and maintaining healthy habits. It seems that the combination of personal and situational factors, taken together, suggest that people who maintain healthy habits are different on selected personal characteristics than their less healthy counterparts. People with healthy habits are more devoted to taking control of their lives than people who perceive themselves as victims of life's events. While this is not to suggest that traditional personality traits embedded throughout the psychology literature (e.g., neuroticism, stability, dominant, extraversion, introversion, trait anxiety) are useless in explaining actions that are intended to maintain health and enhance quality of life. However, certain thought patterns and dispositions seem to help explain why we differ in our desire to invest time and energy in maintaining a healthy lifestyle.

Remaining in control of our quality of life (i.e., happiness, health, lack of disease and sickness) and living a life consistent with our values, the central theme of this book, are desirable. In the next chapter, we examine personal qualities that inhibit good health.

References

Clough, P., Earle, K., & Sewell, D. (2002). Mental toughness: The concept and its measurement. In I. Cockerill (Ed.), *Solutions in sport psychology* (pp. 32–45). London, England: Thomson.

Hagger, M.S., & Chatzisarantis, N.L.D. (Eds., 2007). *Intrinsic motivation and self- determination in exercise and sport*. Champaign, IL: Human Kinetics.

Jones, G., Hanton, S., & Connaughton, D. (2007). A framework of mental toughness in the world's best performers. *The Sport Psychologist, 21*, 243–264.

Roberts, G.C., & Treasure, D. C. (2012). *Advances in motivation in sport and exercise*. Champaign, IL: Human Kinetics.

Rosenbaum, M. (Ed., 1990). *Learned resourcefulness on coping skills, self-control, and adaptive behavior*. New York: Springer.

18

PERSONAL QUALITIES THAT *INHIBIT* HEALTHY HABITS

The previous chapter covered the personal characteristics that promote healthy habits and adhering to desirable actions, such as exercise, proper dieting and nutrition, and effective stress management. Other personal characteristics, however, are *impediments* to developing and adhering to healthy habits. Some of these characteristics and traits require psychotherapy or some other form of counseling because they constitute or border on mental illness. Sometimes people behave in a self-destructive manner that can only be explained by engaging in therapy with a credentialed mental health professional. This section addresses some of these personal factors and traits.

Dysfunctional (emotional) eating and obesity: The American Dietetic Association (ADA, 2009) defines *obesity* as a condition characterized by excess accumulation of fat stores, equal to being at least 30 pounds overweight. While managing fat stores is the key to preventing or overcoming obesity, at times people cannot control their eating habits—at least not without therapy. As the ADA contends, fat stores can only occur by a change in energy intake, energy output, efficiency of energy use, or a combination of any of these components. While many overweight individuals rationalize their overweight or obese condition as "genetic" ("My whole family is overweight, so I can't do anything about it") or feel vindicated by their personal care provider ("My doctor says I'm healthy so I do not need to worry about my weight"), the ADA claims there have been only a limited number of obesity cases identified as being directly caused by a single gene mutation.

There are several types of dysfunctional eating patterns. Three of these, however, seem to be most prominent and strongly influence health, emotion, and quality of life: disordered eating, eating disorders, and emotional eating. The Disconnected Values Model is more effective if these areas of psychopathology (mental illness) are diagnosed and properly treated.

Disordered eating may be defined on a continuum from eating disorders (e.g., anorexia nervosa, bulimia nervosa) to preoccupation with weight and restrictive eating. The condition of disordered eating is often and wrongly used interchangeably with the condition *eating disorders*. For example, a *disordered eating* pattern is a habitual reaction to life situations, such as stress or wanting to appear thin for a particular event. An *eating disorder*, on the other hand, is a mental illness, such as anorexia nervosa (self-starvation) or bulimia (binge and purge or vomit food recently consumed). In addition, disordered eating is not usually accompanied by frequent thoughts of food, eating, and a preoccupation with remaining thin to enhance one's physical appearance.

Persons with eating disorders, on the other hand, have compulsive thoughts of food, eating, and one's body. Another difference between disordered eating and eating disorders is the extent of sickness associated with each. Disordered eating may lead to transient weight changes and nutritional problems, but rarely are there major medical complications. Eating disorders, on the other hand, often lead to serious medical problems; in fact, approximately 10% of persons diagnosed with an eating disorder will die from this mental illness (Williams, 2006).

Depression: Depression is a mood disorder that ranges from mild to severe and, if diagnosed by a mental health professional, may reflect mental illness. Most authors in this area depict depression as a "depressed" (chronically unhappy or dissatisfied) mood or a loss of interest or pleasure in all or most activities *for at least two consecutive weeks*. Symptoms of depression include loss of appetite, weight loss or gain, disturbance of sleep, disruption of psychomotor skills, decreased energy, feeling worthless, guilt, poor concentration, and thoughts of suicide (Leith, 1998). Over 70 studies across different age groups and both genders have shown that aerobic exercise reduces clinical (severe) depression.

Measuring and counseling for depression is reserved for mental health professionals who are trained and licensed by their respective states to help clients overcome this condition. Professionals with the titles "consultants" or "coaches" who are not licensed may have expertise in changing unhealthy habits and providing instruction to clients, but they must not provide formal counseling to deal with clients' mental health issues. It is no wonder, however, that persons suffering from clinical (chronic) depression are *less* likely to practice healthy habits than their nondepressed counterparts.

Anxiety: Anxiety consists of feelings of threat or worry about a future event or situation. It can occur in either acute (short-term bouts) or chronic form (long-term, persistent attacks). *Clinical anxiety*, a possible form of mental illness if diagnosed by a mental health professional, leads to changes in a person's thoughts and actions. This condition may occur even without some initiating event and when the response is disproportionate and unmanageable. Ironically, anxiety is actually healthy, even potentially lifesaving, under certain conditions (e.g., crossing the street and looking both ways, being cautious when walking down a flight of stairs, walking carefully on snow or ice, competing cautiously against the opposing sports team). Anxiety, however, can be a disorder and debilitating to normal thinking, quality of life, happiness, and general mental well-being.

Perhaps not surprisingly, clinical anxiety leads to a preoccupation with unpleasant thoughts, lack of energy, and poor health. Behavioral strategies that combat debilitating forms of anxiety have been studied extensively and form part of an "action plan" in the Disconnected Values Model.

Neurotic Perfectionism: Perfectionism is a multidimensional concept that can impede the development and adherence to healthy habits. Perfectionism may be viewed as both desirable (adaptive) or undesirable (maladaptive or neurotic). Adaptive perfectionism reflects setting reasonably challenging and achievable goals, having high personal standards, possessing a strong desire to excel, being self-forgiving of one's own mistakes, modifying standards in accordance with situational factors, striving for success in achievement settings, and having enhanced levels of motivation (Ellis, 2002).

Neurotic perfectionism, on the other hand, a concept relevant to this section, describes the tendency to set excessively high standards; be overly self-critical; and be extensively influenced by the approval of significant others, such as parents, teachers, peers, and sports coaches. Individuals who are characterized as maladaptive perfectionists tend to exhibit exaggerated expectations, have a high fear of failure, and are less capable of coping with challenging situations. Perhaps not surprisingly, then, perfectionism has been traditionally perceived as negative, also referred to as undesirable, abnormal, neurotic, maladaptive, or dysfunctional. Maladaptive perfectionism is a primary component of various psychopathologies (Ellis, 2002). It is not surprising, therefore, that this thinking pattern is self-destructive because the intended goal—in this case, changing a bad habit for a better one—is either not attainable or will lead to certain dropout when experiencing the first "failure." Typical self-talk for this person might be: "If I fail to floss for a week I may as well stop trying," or "If I am too ill (injured) to exercise for a week I may as well quit and not even try."

Irrational thinking: "I don't deserve to be healthy" or "I absolutely must have perfect teeth and no cavities" are examples of this disposition, which is considered psychopathological. The late clinical psychologist, Dr. Albert Ellis, separates the normal desire to have or believe something from the abnormal *dire necessity*, in which one must have something. He says that "failing to perform well or perfectly well and succeeding in performing badly or imperfectly will likely get you less of what you want; less approval from others; and make you less likely to be safe from disease, harm, and death. . . . Your wish or desire to have a sense of self-efficacy is a rational belief not an irrational belief" (Ellis, 2002, p. 219). Strong preferences, he believes, often leave few alternative choices of equal valence. Strong preferences leave little room for alternative choices or at least equally satisfying ones. It implied that because alternatives don't exist, we must have strong preferences fulfilled. "Raising your 'want' to a 'necessity' is your irrationality," he says (p. 220). It's rational to *want* to win the game; however, it is irrational thinking to *absolutely must* win, and the person believes there are horrible consequences of losing or not obtaining what was desired.

With respect to health and happiness, people are more likely to feel stressed when they insist that stress *must not* exist, as opposed to effectively coping with the inevitability of experiencing a stressful event or situation. It is one thing to feel disappointment, regret, and frustration when people's weak desires are thwarted, such as failing to sleep soundly despite performing the right presleep rituals. However, it is quite another thing when people's strong desires are thwarted, leading to absolutistic "musts" and "demands" and unhealthy feelings of anxiety, depression, rage, and self-pity. The consequence of irrational beliefs is often giving up, dropping out, nonadherence, and lacking the motivation to overcome obstacles and feel driven to meet goals. Irrational thinking is unhealthy, mentally and physically. Separate "desires," "wishes," and "wants" from "absolutely must have." Accept imperfection and maintain reasonable needs and expectations.

Low self-confidence, self-efficacy, and self-esteem: These concepts are grouped together because of their similar features, especially in the real world. However, they are also different. Self-confidence is a *general* feeling, perception, or belief that the person has the capability to be successful in performing a task or meeting a goal. Self-efficacy (SE), on the other hand, combines confidence with self-expectations. Self-efficacy is a person's belief about being able to execute a specific task successfully to obtain a certain predetermined outcome. Self-efficacy beliefs are not judgments about one's skills but rather are judgments of what one can accomplish with those skills. Thus, self-efficacy beliefs do not reflect a person's feelings about what he or she can do but rather what the person has already done. Thus, persons who possess self-doubt about their ability to adopt a new healthy habit ("I've already tried an exercise program and dropped out; why try it again?") will more likely avoid attempting a new habit or discontinue it after they have started and revert to their previous unhealthy lifestyle.

It is against human nature to maintain participation in an activity in which individuals perceive their performance as incompetent or failing to meet their own or others' expectations. Therefore, building self-confidence/efficacy in attempting to begin and maintain new habits is challenging and must be experienced slowly and successfully.

With respect to general health, if people lack self-confidence/efficacy, they will likely feel incapable of experiencing superior health-related outcomes (e.g., more energy, positive mood, favorable results from medical tests). The objective of every worker in the health care industry, including fitness and nutrition coaches, is to provide instruction and positive feedback to build people's self-confidence and efficacy about their ability to maintain proper healthy habits.

While self-efficacy is relatively low at the early stages of starting new healthy habits, SC and SE increase dramatically as the person inserts the new habit into his or her daily rituals. What is unknown is whether SE causes a person to adopt exercise as a lifestyle ritual or if continued exercise increases SE. No doubt the two processes interact. They are both the cause and the outcome of maintaining regular healthy habits.

Self-esteem: Self-esteem reflects how we feel about who we are, that is, the extent to which we value ourselves. Self-esteem consists of evaluating how well the self is doing, both in specific areas and in general. It is a concept used interchangeably with these related terms: self-regard, self-respect, self-acceptance, and self-worth. Self-esteem is multidimensional, including physical, religious, social, intellectual, and sport sources of both constructs. It has been considered a personality trait but at the same time is open to change through age, experience, skill level, and learning (McKay & Fanning, 2000).

Of particular importance in the present context is that people with low self-esteem are more likely to be pessimistic about their future health and being able to adopt new, healthier habits successfully. Moreover, because people with low self-esteem have low evaluations of their skills and potential for change, they are less likely to be optimistic about the outcomes of their attempts at improved health. Moreover, people with low self-esteem are less likely to feel that they deserve better health and, therefore, tend to drop out of health interventions more quickly than people who are highly optimistic about their future health and adopting routines that improve health.

Poor self-control: Self-control refers to a person's conscious decision and action to plan and maintain thoughts, emotions, and behaviors toward reaching desirable goals, even after encountering events that might impede these processes. Self-control behaviors are controlled by deliberate cognitive processes that are under the person's voluntary control (Rosenbaum, 1990). A good example of self-control in developing healthy habits is time management.

Perhaps the main reason "not enough time" is a primary reason for not exercising is the lack of self-control skills. Individuals with high self-control skills plan their days and set aside time (i.e., day of the week, time of day, types of exercises) devoted to maintaining an exercise routine or any other healthy habit. High-quality sleep, for instance, is more likely if the person goes to bed at a consistent hour. Lack of self-control skills results in lack of planning of one's day, inconsistent and dysfunctional behavior patterns, and lack of attention to maintaining healthy habits.

Lack of proper self-regulation (SR): SR consist of executing a task that allows performers to control or direct their own activity through self-imposed rules or regulations. The goal of SR is to adapt behaviors to different circumstances, situations, or surroundings.

To Zimmerman (1986), SR consists of three subcomponents, each of which has implications in exercise settings. The *metacognitive* component consists of planning, organizing, self-instructing, self-monitoring, and self-evaluating at various stages during performance. The *motivational* component consists of performers perceiving themselves as competent, autonomous, and confident, or self-efficacious. Finally, the *behavioral* component reflects selecting, structuring, and creating environments that optimize goal-directed behavior, that is, helping the individual to achieve predetermined goals.

The behavioral component of SR consists of acting at a given location and environment under specific conditions; using equipment; and obtaining instruction, if needed, to achieve personal goals. Keeping records of performance outcomes is also part of self-regulation as a way to self-monitor progress or detect deficiencies as sources of personal motivation and competence. The lack of proper self-monitoring is referred to as self-regulation failure.

Sadly, it is not uncommon to "drop the ball" when it comes to successful self-regulation. SR is based on the premise that the individual is both self-motivated and capable of engaging independently in tasks that will lead to achieving goal-directed performance outcomes. If, for instance, we brush our teeth and floss "regularly," it is far less likely we will suffer from dental and periodontal disease than if we did not perform these tasks. If an athlete engages in the proper training regimen and practices the requisite sport skills, performance success under competitive conditions is far more likely than if practice and other game preparation are neglected. The concept of SR failure means that a person does not carry out the cognitive and behavioral strategies that are necessary for task success; goals are not met.

Examples of SR failure related to health behavior abound in our culture. Dentists tell us to floss our teeth, dieticians urge us to eat breakfast and not overeat near bedtime, and we all know the benefits of regular exercise and other forms of physical activity. And yet, many of us fail at each of these preferred habits. SR means we make a conscious decision to develop habits that have desirable outcomes, including improved health, more energy, slower aging, improved mood, and reduced chance of mental illness. While all of us self-regulate certain behavior patterns, sometimes those behaviors are self-destructive and unhealthy.

While many of these undesirable characteristics impede practicing healthy habits, especially over a lifetime, each can be changed with professional treatment. Even personality traits, while permanent and always present, can alter their effects on behavior. A person with heightened trait anxiety, for example, can learn anxiety management skills to help regulate the frequency and intensity of anxious thoughts and emotions. Maintaining healthy habits, such as physical activity, high-quality sleep, stress management, and proper eating habits, will result in reduced anxiety and other unpleasant thoughts and emotions. Healthier behaviors are likely to result. An important focus of the DVM is to facilitate this process.

References

American Dietetic Association. (2009). Position of the American Dietetic Association: Weight management. *Journal of the American Dietetic Association, 109*, 330–346.

Ellis, A. (2002). The role of irrational beliefs in perfectionism. In G.L. Flett & P.L. Hewitt (Eds.), *Perfectionism: Theory, research, and treatment* (pp. 217–229).

Leith, L. (1998). *Exercising your way to better mental health*. Morgantown, WV: Fitness Information Technology.
McKay, M., & Fanning, P. (2000). *Self-esteem* (3rd ed.). Oakland, CA: New Harbinger.
Rosenbaum, M. (1990). Role of learned resourcefulness in self-control of health behavior. In M. Rosenbaum (Ed.), *Learned resourcefulness on coping skills, self-control, and adaptive behavior* (pp. 3–30). New York: Springer Publishing Company.
Williams, M. (2006). *Nutrition for health, fitness, and sport* (5th ed.). New York: McGraw-Hill.

19

ROLE OF SPIRITUALITY IN MAINTAINING A HEALTHY LIFESTYLE

> "Don't you know that you yourselves are God's temple and that God's Spirit lives in you? If anyone destroys God's temple, God will destroy him; for God's temple is sacred, and you are that temple"
>
> (I Corinthians 3:16–17)

> "Your body is a temple of the Holy Spirit within you, which you have from God"
>
> (I Corinthians 6:19).

For a secular book and reader audience, this chapter may seem controversial for some readers. However, 93% of U.S. adults believe in a higher power (Levin, 2001), and health plays an important role in the spiritual (and religious) life of many individuals. This chapter is *not* about describing the healing powers of religious beliefs or having a spiritual life. The focus of this chapter is to examine the evidence that links one's spirituality with health, the role of faith in maintaining healthy habits, and implications for practitioners to include spirituality in properly using the DVM for people of faith. Should spiritual and religious leader become involved in promoting healthy habits among their followers? For selected individuals who believe in a higher power, the answer is "absolutely," according to numerous studies. First, however, we need to define relevant terms.

Differences between Religion and Spirituality

While the terms *spirituality* and *religion* are sometimes used interchangeably in the literature, they differ markedly. If a person claims to be "spiritual but not religious," he or she likely believes in a higher power but have no formal ties to a specific religion. Levin (2001) draws the differences between spirituality and religion, which form an important issue when working with particular clients. Religion, he contends, denotes: (a) organized religious institutions and buildings for worship, (b) a scholarly field of study, and (c) an area of life that deals with issues related to the person's spirit and matters of personal concern. "Practicing religion" or "being religious" refers to a person's behaviors, attitudes, beliefs, and experiences that involve this domain of life. Thus, religion consists of a connection between humans and a higher power (e.g., God, Mohammad, Buddha).

Similarly, Koenig (2008) defines religion as "a system of beliefs and practices observed by a community supported by rituals that acknowledge, worship, communicate with, or approach the Sacred . . . (or) God in Western cultures" (p. 11). Religion typically offers a moral code of conduct agreed upon by community members, who attempt to live according to that code.

Spirituality, on the other hand, "refers to a state of being that is acquired through religious devotion, piety, and observance" (Levin, 2001, p. 9). Spirituality is the ultimate goal and a subset of religion; it consists of a union or connection with God or the divine. Spirituality is something to be attained through religious participation. In more recent years, however, spirituality has taken on a new meaning. To Levin, spirituality consists of private religious expression such as meditation and feelings of oneness with nature, referred to as "secular transcendent experiences" (p. 10). In the more contemporary definition, spirituality is the larger phenomenon, and religion is reserved for more organized religious activity.

Koenig (2008) contends that "many people find spirituality through religion or thorough a personal relationship with the divine" (p. 13). Others, however, may find spirituality through a connection to nature, through music and the arts, through a set of values, or through attempting to discover scientific truth. Spirituality is a personal relationship with a higher power, and religion is the community and institutional aspects, or the expression, of spirituality.

One additional area related to practicing one's faith that has grown increasingly contentious in recent years is the "disconnect," or inconsistency, between a person's religious/spiritual beliefs about a relationship with a higher power and his or her unhealthy lifestyle, an issue that will be addressed in greater depth later in the chapter because it forms the basis of the DVM (Anshel, 2008).

Spirituality and Healthy Habits

The spiritual person is not immune from the health problems derived from an unhealthy lifestyle.

One potentially powerful source of health behavior change that has been neglected by researchers and practitioners is the inclusion of spiritualty and spiritual leaders. Spiritual leaders are among the most credible persons who influence a person of faith's thoughts, emotions, and actions.

Dr. Harold Koenig, in his book, *Medicine, Religion, and Health: Where Science and Spirituality Meet* (2008), concluded that spirituality was strongly associated with superior health outcomes. Koenig found, for example, that blood pressure and rates of stroke and cognitive impairment were each highly correlated with spirituality. Specific measures included religious service attendance, frequency of prayer, and strength of belief in a higher power. But perhaps more important in Koenig's findings are the clinical applications of religious and spiritual beliefs in promoting health behavior. Although not always acknowledged by spiritual leaders, messages related to maintaining healthy habits are common throughout most spiritual texts.

Scripture and a Healthy Lifestyle

Most religious texts are replete with passages that extol the virtues of living a healthy lifestyle. One of the most powerful passages in the Biblical narrative concerning our perspective on our bodies is found in 1 Corinthians 6:19–20 "Do you not know that your body is a temple of the Holy Spirit, who is in you, whom you have received from God? You are not your own; you were bought at a price. Therefore, honor God with your body." Perhaps if spiritually enlightened individuals adopted this perspective for our bodies, we would begin to make appropriate decisions that directly influence our physical and spiritual health.

Given the virtual mandate by religious texts to be stewards of our "temple" (body), it is surprising that so many people of faith who: (a) profess to a strong belief in a higher power, (b) become members of spiritual institutions, and (c) regularly attend services and other spiritual programs also choose to engage in self-destructive habits that compromise their health, energy, and mental status.

EXAMPLES OF SCRIPTURAL PASSAGES THAT PROMOTE HEALTHY LIFESTYLE

* "Let us purify ourselves from everything that contaminate body and spirit, perfecting holiness out of reverence for God." (II Corinthians 7:1)
* "How much more so am I required to scrub and scour myself, having been created in the image and likeness of God, as it is written 'For in the image of God He made human beings.'" (Genesis 9:6; Leviticus Rabbah 34:3)
* "So whether you eat or drink, or whatever you do, do it all for the glory of God." (I Corinthians 10:31)
* "Do you not know that you are the temple of God and that the Spirit of God dwells in you?" (I Corinthians 3:16)

* "It is not good to eat too much honey, nor is it honorable to seek one's own honor. Like a city whose walls are broken down is a man (or woman) who lacks self-control." (Proverbs 25:27–28)
* "The good man eats to live while the evil man lives to eat." (Proverbs 13:25)
* "Do not join those who drink too much wine or gorge themselves on meat, for drunkards and gluttons become poor, and drowsiness clothes them in rags." (Proverbs 23: 20–21)

There are over 56 passages in the Old and New Testaments that depict a healthy lifestyle, as shown by the following examples.

For a person of faith, there is probably no individual who has more credibility and influence on that person's thoughts, emotions, beliefs, and actions than his or her religious leader. Acknowledging the importance of religious leaders and their use of effective interventions that favorably influence health behavior has been surprisingly neglected in the research and practitioner literature. It is apparent that while most spiritual texts condone a healthy lifestyle, spiritual leaders do not provide substance on this topic through sermon content and their respective religious programs. Instead, they fail to address a culture of wellness and the mandate, clearly articulated in Scripture, to develop and maintain healthy habits among members and worshipers (Young & Koopsen, 2005).

Contradictions between Spirituality and Unhealthy Living

This section is at the heart of the Disconnected Values Model because of the inconsistency exhibited between spirituality (and religion) and certain habits that can harm health and reduce energy and quality of life. The doctrines of many faiths offer moral and practical guidance concerning ways to attain, maintain, and recover physical, mental, emotional, and spiritual health. While these laws differ among individuals and religions, they share the common goal of helping to ensure that people of faith have a long and productive life. Indeed, the health-related benefits of following a strong spiritual life have been documented in numerous studies (see Levin, 2001 for a review).

Here is the main disconnect that therapists and coaches need to help their clients identify: It is bewildering—and wrong—for a person to proclaim a strong spiritual identity and observe the customs of their faith and yet not maintain healthy behavior patterns that would improve his or her devotion to a higher power. The consequence is less energy and poorer general health toward practicing one's faith to a higher power. In addition, despite knowledge of their religious or spiritual text, these individuals appear to ignore or discount the importance of many passages that lend strong support for maintaining a healthy lifestyle. Thus, it would seem logical that spiritual use of the DVM should include the link between meaningful Scriptural messages and a strong commitment to making healthy lifestyle choices.

Is it possible that people of faith may actually feel *less* control of their ability to maintain healthy habits because "my life is in 'His' hands?" To what extent do a person's spiritual practices and beliefs dictate their health-related behavior patterns, a process called *spiritual health* (Holt & McClure, 2006)? Are people healthier if they surrender control of their life to a higher power, as opposed to people who take control of their long-term health and destiny? Do firmly held spiritual beliefs and practices result in feeling more responsible for one's health? Or, conversely, do people who surrender self-control to a higher power and maintain habits not take into account the findings of medical research or the advice of their personal physician?

To Young and Koopsen (2005), it is hypocritical for those who profess their devotion to a higher power to maintain unhealthy habits that will lead to illness, disease, lack of energy, and a shortened lifespan. We should all feel responsible, they contend, for what we accomplish in life, including being responsible for one's own health, but we should also feel responsible for one's own quality of life, perhaps with spiritual support.

Physical and Mental Health Benefits

The relationship between spiritual practices and physical health has been examined in the literature. It is well known that individuals who practice a strong spirituality experience superior health outcomes as opposed to their nonreligious counterparts (George, Larson, Koenig, & McCullough, 2000; Levin, 2001). In their review of related literature, for example, Koenig (1999), Marks (2005), and Levin (2001) concluded that religious practitioners were more likely to have healthier lifestyles, a stronger sense of well-being and life satisfaction, stronger immune systems, and greater lifespan than their nonreligious counterparts.

Several factors have been shown to help explain the benefits of behavior patterns that promote good health among those who practice a spiritual or religious lifestyle. One of these factors is increased social support (e.g., religious leaders, family, members of the religious institution). Surrounding oneself with individuals who provide support, understanding, and motivation is referred to as the *buffering hypothesis* (Kinney, Bloor, Dudley, Millikan, Marshall, Martin, & Sandler, 2003). Individuals with a strong social support system are healthier and suffer from less mental illness and disease (Commerford & Reznikoff, 1996).

Another factor that links spirituality with good health is the propensity of more spiritual persons to engage in fewer unhealthy behaviors because of content in religious or spiritual texts. Spirituality empowers individuals to take personal responsibility for their health by experiencing reduced frequency and intensity of perceived stress, using effective coping skills that include a strong spiritual component, following superior dietary habits dictated by various texts, experiencing positive emotions as part of spiritual practice, and gaining improved mental health (Koenig, 1999). Musick (1996) found in his study of the elderly that frequent participation in devotional activities was significantly and positively related to perceived good health. While the act of prayer appears to be one mechanism that enhances health, there is another perspective on the religion-health connection, given the evidence of an obesity epidemic in the United States and elsewhere.

The results of numerous studies have reported favorable effects of spirituality and religious practice on health (Atchley, 1997; Ferraro & Albrecht-Jensen, 1991). The likely reasons for these benefits include the use of prayer and spirituality as a form of coping with stress, reduced use of addictive drugs, reduced use of nicotine and excessive alcohol, and elevated positive mood state. In addition to improved physical health, there is also a similar improvement in spiritual and mental health (Holt & McClure, 2006). Perhaps the most salient forbidden unhealthy habit mentioned repeatedly in the Scripture is gluttony.

Gluttony is the object of disdain in many faiths. The sin of gluttony is a strong contributing factor to premature deaths of thousands of individuals. To Colbert (2002), Christians do not discuss gluttony because they do not think of themselves as gluttons. Gluttony has been divorced from obesity in their minds so that it becomes merely a health issue rather than a spiritual and moral one. The contradiction between excessive eating and maintaining a spiritual life borders on hypocrisy and yet may represent an opportunity for health care providers and consultants to cite spiritual messages to selected clients to encourage healthy lifestyle choices. Gluttony forms the primary cause of obesity among people of faith, Colbert contends.

The Bible condemns overindulgence in many things, including health-related issues. Proverbs 23:20–21 says: "Don't associate with those who drink too much wine, or with those who gorge themselves on meat." Gluttony is placed in the same category as other sinful behavior. Yet, while most religious leaders denounce the use of excessive alcohol, many tend not to speak up about the sin of overeating even though the lack of self-control is usually the root of both problems (Cline & Ferraro, 2006).

Spector (1996) contends that nearly every religious and spiritual person espouses beliefs that govern behavior concerning health, disease, and death. Beliefs require certain health behaviors, while others forbid certain behaviors related to health or medical care. Many doctrines or teachings of faith offer moral and practical guidance about how to attain, maintain, or recover physical health and well-being. Just as with refraining from cigarettes or alcohol or overeating, religious affiliation may prevent or lay pathogenic (illness-making) changes and have long-term benefits for physical and mental functioning and health. Another area that might explain the role of religious and spiritual practice on health is the extent to which a person feels in control of his or her health as opposed to a higher power in control of health and well-being, a process called surrendering style.

Gall et al. (2005) speculate that unhealthy behavior patterns among religious practitioners could be due to their *surrendering style*. To Gall et al., "a surrendering style involves an active decision to release personal control to God over those aspects of a situation that fall outside of one's control" (p. 92). Therefore, the person believes that "God is now in charge of the situation" (p. 92). For believers in a higher power, this disposition promotes spiritual well-being and a deepened sense of faith, especially under conditions of high stress. The authors do not suggest that a person's surrender style gives him or her license to engage in a carelessly unhealthy lifestyle because, after all, "God is in control." However, it is plausible to speculate that for some individuals, a strong religious surrender style provides the incentive to maintain behavior patterns that medical science would consider unhealthy, such as lack of exercise and poor dietary habits.

A person's surrender style, in some cases, may explain their relatively passive attitude toward taking responsibility for maintaining healthy habits. This is an issue of particular importance to health professionals. As Omartian (1996) contends in relation to the common health problem of obesity, "The biggest problem with excess weight is not whether God still loves you. He does, and so do other people. Nor is the biggest problem whether you look good in your clothes. The most important thing is whether you're going to be incapacitated by fat-related diseases and die prematurely" (pp. 89–90).

The Neglected Role of Religious Institutions on Health Behavior Change

Health care professionals—therapists, fitness coaches, dieticians, nurses, among others—should attempt to recruit staff in relation to health behavior change among people of faith. To people of faith, arguably no one has more credibility than their religious or spiritual leader. How can these leaders assist others in reducing unhealthy behavior patterns and embracing the plethora of scriptural passages and other narrative that pontificate the virtues of leading a healthy lifestyle? How can religious and spiritual leaders address the apparent disconnect between one's religious or spiritual practices and the lack of self-awareness about practicing healthy habits?

The Role of Spiritual Leaders in Promoting and Modeling Healthy Habits

If the health care professional wishes to recruit a spiritual leader to assist clients in changing health behavior, here are some important considerations.

(1) Spiritual leaders need to look at themselves and determine if they are the proper models for health behavior change. Should improving one's health and developing proper habits start with them?
(2) They must encourage their institution members—and other members of the community, when given the opportunity—to have discipline in all areas of

their lives. Topics related to healthy living need to be addressed without fear of offending attendees.
(3) Congregations should expect their leaders to encourage them to make lifestyle changes that will ultimately bring glory to the higher power they may worship or some other higher power to whom they feel accountable. Religious and spiritual leaders must stop being intimidated by the risk of losing members by offending anyone (Colbert, 2002).

Perhaps the most serious *obstacle* to health behavior change among spiritual people is their refusal to take responsibility for their health and their willingness to surrender control of their lives to a higher power. If "it's all in God's hands," why be concerned about making healthy lifestyle choices? Keep in mind the concept of "free will" that consists of taking responsibility for one's health and well-being because ultimately each person is in control of his or her destiny based on one's own freedom and decision. The lack of perceived self-control is contrary to the concept of free will; even if a higher power gave us life and guides our footsteps, it remains our responsibility to be a steward of our bodies. To quote Scripture as an example, "God works within us to will his holy spirit and the free will to have the desire to create balance in our life—and the will to act on that desire" (Philippians NIV 2:13).

Omartian (1996) contends that "The main reason to exercise is for your health. Without good health you cannot do all that the Lord has for you do to and you cannot be all the Lord wants you to be." (p. 117). In support of the need to exert greater self-control over one's health and future destiny from a spiritual context, Koenig (1999) asserts, "The world's religions encourage healthy living. . . . All established religions discourage . . . any habit or activity harmful to the human body, which has traditionally been viewed as sacred, created in the image of God" (p. 72). As Levin (2001) concludes, "All (spiritual groups) endorse the idea that we ought to take care of our bodies and not act in ways that are reckless and endanger our health" (p. 41).

The spiritual leader is uniquely qualified and credible to provide others with inspirational and motivational reasons to maintain a healthy lifestyle. This includes the capability of learning and carrying out the DVM program. Few individuals possess more respect, credibility, and integrity in fulfilling the spiritual life of people who believe in a higher power. The ability to promote the concept of *free will* in living a life consistent with one's values is consistent with Scripture. It is the primary mission of religious leaders to help others—and themselves—to lead a high quality of life, both physically and spiritually, which includes a devotion to a higher power.

Creating Health as Sermon Themes

Perhaps the strongest influence of spiritual leaders on the thoughts, emotions, and actions of others, including religious service attendees, is the leader's sermon. Health-related themes are needed more frequently and communicated more passionately that extol the virtues of maintaining a healthy lifestyle, citing spiritual text (e.g., Scripture, the Koran, the Talmud) to reinforce main issues. Thus, maintaining unhealthy habits that lead to obesity and poor physical conditioning is a stewardship issue that spiritual leaders must be willing to address to their followers and congregations.

Clinical Applications

I asked the Corporate Executive Officer of a corporate wellness center in Orlando, Florida, why his program does not include or address "faith" as an integral part of one's belief system, nor include content about the role of religion or spirituality in maintaining a healthy lifestyle. He responded that it was important that the program remain secular and not "impose" faith as a value or a strategy that is intended to remove unhealthy habits and promote a healthy lifestyle.

Koenig (2008) has a different view of what health professionals and medical practitioners should and should not include when administering faith-based counseling. He offers a list of "dos" and "do not's" related to the application of spirituality in patient/client care.

In Favor of the Following Faith-based Strategies

Consider patient spirituality or religiosity. Many patients are religious, with a vast majority who believe in a higher power. Many of these individuals would like to have faith included in their health care. Spiritual needs should be recognized and addressed by their health care providers.

Spirituality and religion influence patients' ability to cope with illness. The ability to cope with illness, injury, or poor health provides additional incentive to experience proper self-care; spiritual individuals are more likely to adhere to planned medical treatment.

Religious beliefs and practices may influence medical outcomes. Stress has an adverse effect on the success of medical treatments and can compromise the immune system. Expression of religious or spiritual beliefs among persons who believe in a higher power reduces stress and, therefore, improves physical, mental, and emotional health. Having a religious or spiritual leader lead prayer for persons of faith enhances mental health and, ostensibly, medical outcomes.

Patients are often isolated from other sources of spiritual help. If a patient is hospitalized or experiences a medical "event" away from his or her faith community or spiritual leader, the patient is more likely to feel isolated and alone, which will impeded recovery. In addition, clergy may not be able to visit all patients or be limited in the frequency of such visits.

Spiritual or religious beliefs and rituals may conflict with or influence patients' medical decisions. Clinicians need to know how a person's beliefs and related rituals influence the type of care that the patient/client wants and expects. Prayer may or may not be appropriate and included in a session.

Spiritual and religious beliefs influence patient health care in the community or after he/she leaves the hospital or doctor's office. Health care providers need to know what type of support is available to the patient/client when leaving the health care or exercise/wellness facility. Are clients on their own and isolated, or is there a social support network available? Are institutions that offer facilities, equipment, or reduced membership costs at local fitness clubs available?

Not in Favor of the Following Faith-based Actions

Koenig (2008) strongly suggests that medical and health practitioners *not* do the following with respect to including a religious or spiritual component in their practice.

"Prescribe" spirituality or religion. According to Koenig (2008), "health professionals should not prescribe (spirituality or) religion to non-religious/non-spiritual patients or actively proselytize" (p. 169). It is unethical to coerce someone or induce guilt about a particular belief system or behavior pattern, particularly when the person is ill or either physically or emotionally weak.

Record the patient's/client's spiritual history. If the patient/client is not religious and feels uncomfortable or resists questioning about his or her spirituality or religious background or practice, discontinue this type of questioning immediately.

Pray with patients. Medical and health practitioners should avoid praying with their patients/clients unless patients ask. This is an especially relevant issue, Koenig contends, if the patient's religion or spirituality differs from that of the practitioner.

Provide spiritual counseling. Health professionals without proper training should not usually provide spiritual counsel or religious advice to clients/patients. Spiritual needs can be very complex and interact with psychological and social issues.

Argue about religious and spiritual issues. Health practitioners should not argue or debate with patients or clients about their spiritual or religious beliefs, even if those beliefs conflict with medical or health care. Some spiritual or religious organizations, for example, require certain attire or followers must avoid members of the opposite sex in health or exercise settings.

Institutions that include a spiritual component possess enormous influence on the behaviors of community members, participants, and worshipers. To date, spiritual leaders may want to consider citing spiritual or religious text in pontificating the virtues of living a healthy lifestyle that is consistent with their deepest values and beliefs, including faith.

As Koenig (2008) recommends, "integrating spirituality into patient care should be a priority because so many medical patients have spiritual needs, spiritual conflicts, or derive comfort from religious beliefs and traditions, this makes a strong argument for training health professionals to assess, respect, and make accommodations for patients' spiritual beliefs and practices" (p. 172).

References

Anshel, M. H. (2008). The Disconnected Values Model: Intervention strategies for health behavior change. *Journal of Clinical Sport Psychology, 2*, 357–380.

Atchley, R. C. (1997). The subjective importance of being religious and its effect on health and morale 14 years later. *Journal of Aging Studies, 11*, 131–141.

Cline, K.M.C., & Ferraro, K.F. (2006). Does religion increase the prevalence and incidence of obesity in adulthood? *Journal for the Scientific Study of Religion, 45, 269–281.*

Colbert, D. (2002) *What would Jesus eat? The ultimate program for eating well, feeling great, and living longer.* Nashville, TN: Thomas Nelson.

Commerford, M.C., & Reznikoff, M. (1996). Relationship of religion and perceived social support to self-esteem and depression in nursing home residents. *Journal of Psychology, 130*, 141–151.

Ferraro, K. F., & Albrecht-Jensen, C. M. (1991). Does religion influence adult health? *Journal for the Scientific Study of Religion, 30*, 193–202.

Gall, T.L., Charbonneau, C., Clarke, N.H., Grant, K., Joseph, A., & Shouldice, L. (2005). Understanding the nature and role of spirituality in relation to coping and health: A conceptual framework. *Canadian Psychology, 46*, 88–104.

George, L.K., Larson, D.B., Koenig, H.G., & McCullough, M.E. (2000). Spirituality and health: What we know, what we need to know. *Journal of Social and Clinical Psychology, 19*, 102–116.

Holt, C.L., & McClure, S.M. (2006). Perceptions of the religion-health connection among African American church members. *Qualitative Health Research, 16*, 268–281.

Kinney, A.Y., Bloor, L.E., Dudley, W.N., Millikan, R.C., Marshall, E., Martin, C., & Sandler, R.S. (2003). Roles of religious involvement and social support in the risk of colon cancer among Blacks and Whites. *American Journal of Epidemiology, 158*, 1097–1107.

Koenig, H.G. (1999). *The healing power of faith.* New York: Simon and Schuster.

Koenig, H.G. (2008). *Medicine, religion, and health: Where science and spirituality meet.* West Conshohocken, PA: Templeton Foundation Press.

Levin, J. (2001). *God, faith, and health: Exploring the spirituality-healing connection.* New York: John Wiley & Sons.

Marks, L. (2005). Religion and bio-psycho-social health: A review and conceptual model. *Journal of Religion and Health, 44*, 173–186.

Musick, M.A. (1996). Religion and subjective health among black and white elders. *Journal of Health and Social Behavior, 37*, 221–237.

Omartian, S. (1996). *Greater health God's way.* Eugene, OR: Harvest House.

Spector, R.E. (1996). *Cultural diversity in health and illness* (4th ed.). Stamford, CT: Appleton & Lange.

Young, C., & Koopsen, C. (2005). *Spirituality, health, and healing.* Sudbury, MA: Jones and Bartlett.

20

SAMPLE APPLICATIONS OF THE DISCONNECTED VALUES MODEL

The purpose of this chapter is to propose ways in which the DVM can be applied under different conditions—individual versus group settings, for instance—and client needs and characteristics (e.g., work versus personal issues, health or relationships, secular or spiritual issues). As indicated earlier, the model consists of: (a) a set of cognitive and behavioral strategies that compares a person's most important beliefs, called (core) values, with his or her unhealthy habits; (b) identified inconsistencies, or disconnects, between the person's unhealthy behavioral patterns and his or her values; (c) the client's conclusion, given the costs and consequences of persisting with these unhealthy habits, that the disconnect is unacceptable—with input from the health provider or coach; (d) the client's indication of his or her readiness to embark on an action plan with the coach or therapist, which allows the person to carry out new behaviors to replace negative, unhealthy habits with more desirable routines. The focus of this model is to provide a framework for practitioners (e.g., licensed psychologists, dieticians, exercise/fitness consultants, mental health professionals, lifestyle coaches) to provide clients with the incentive to develop one or more long-term habits that are consistent with their values.

Intended Clients of the DVM

The DVM is intended for young and middle-aged adults, as opposed to children, adolescents, and the elderly, for several reasons. First, it is the adult population with whom this model was conceptualized and validated. Second, unlike adults, children and adolescent age groups do not tend to contemplate the costs and long-term problems, or consequences, associated with unhealthy behaviors, such as lack of exercise and poor nutrition, and their values differ markedly from adults. Third, adults would more likely be compatible with the DVM's components and provided examples than other age groups. For example, limitations in physical health and other ailments or unique sociocultural conditioning may inhibit exercise behavior, particularly among the elderly. Motives for exercising and other healthy habits also differ as a function of age. Exercise, for the purpose of enhancing social interaction, is far more common among the elderly, particularly women, while men generally exercise for health reasons. Restrictions on physical activity due to taking medication, injury, discomfort, and other reasons are another concern that is more common among the elderly. Changes in body weight and improved musculature, on the other hand, would be a primary exercise motive for younger age groups. Finally, age groups have different barriers to exercise habits. The elderly, for instance, are more likely to consider transportation or medication a barrier to regular exercise, while this is less likely among the adult population. Thus, the DVD is intended for the adult population.

The Importance of Values

At the heart of the DVM is values. Values are core beliefs that guide and motivate behavior, and provide standards against which we assess behavior (Rokeach, 1973). Values are more central determinants of behavior than are interests and attitudes (Super, 1995), the latter of which are more situational and derived from a core set of values. In addition, interests, attitudes, and needs are transitory and, once satiated, may not influence behavior. Values, on the other hand, are almost always firmly entrenched and stable; therefore, they transcend situations and guide behavior over a long period of time. Thus, many interests and attitudes are derived from relatively fewer values.

Values are highly relevant to establishing a person's individuality in predicting behavior. For example, a person who values health will tend to develop daily rituals and long-term habits that are intended to enhance health and general well-being. To Hogan and Mookherjee (1981), values are "one of the most distinguishing characteristics motivating human beings; the likely effects of values on human behavior, beliefs, and attitudes are indisputable" (p. 29). The authors contend that values guide behavior and that sharing values with others strongly affects their commitment to sacrifice personal, self-serving needs for the benefit of others (e.g., family members, friends, work colleagues). In the present model (i.e., the DVM), behavior will be influenced by the ability to detect a discord between the individual's values and the negative habit of a sedentary lifestyle and lack of an exercise habit.

Implementing the DVM

Here is the process of health behavior change using each stage of the DVM.

Postulates

The DVM is predicated on two postulates, or predictions, that define self-motivated behavior. These postulates have strong implications toward starting and maintaining an exercise habit, which is often missing from existing exercise intervention research.

Postulate One

Self-motivated behavior reflects a person's deepest values and beliefs about his or her passion, that is, the power of purpose. To establish one's purpose, this question must be answered: "What do I want and how do I propose to obtain it?" Purpose generates the desire to become fully engaged in activities that "really matter" (i.e., consistent with values) in meeting personal goals and future aspirations. This is why people who suffer from various forms of mental illness find it very difficult to implement new routines and to look after their health; they are so consumed by their own survival and negative self-talk that there is little energy remaining for developing and maintaining new, healthier ways of behaving.

Postulate Two

Primary motivators of normal human behavior are: (a) to identify one or more deeply held values; (b) to acknowledge the benefits, costs, and long-term consequences of actions that contradict one's values; (c) to live a life and maintain habits and actions that are consistent with one's values; and (d) to consistently hold ourselves accountable to our values in what we say, feel, and do. Ostensibly, people whose values include health, family, faith, happiness, generosity, and performance excellence, among many other values, should be self-motivated to adopt healthy rituals (e.g., exercise, proper sleep, manage stress and anxiety, avoidance of tobacco products) that are consistent with these values and will likely lead to improved health, energy, and quality of life.

A deeper *sense of purpose* consists of shifting one's attention from attempts to address and fulfill one's own needs and desires to serving and meeting the needs and desires of others. For instance, people who love their partner or family realize they will have more energy, better health (i.e., fewer incidences of illness and lower health care costs), and lead a higher quality of life when meeting the needs of family members. This could be represented by foregoing the use of tobacco products, excessive alcohol intake, improving quality and amount of rest and sleep, and leading a more active lifestyle that includes regular exercise. Perhaps, then, the self-motivated drive to develop an exercise habit rests, at least in part, on recognizing the inconsistency between one's negative and unhealthy habits and one's values, acknowledging the short-term costs and long-term consequences of this/these disconnect(s) and then to institute one or more new, "positive" (healthy) habits that reflect one's values (Anshel, 2013).

The DVM is based on the interaction between the practitioner and the client. The interaction reflects receiving information (e.g., facing the truth about who you are and how you live), self-reflection (e.g., acknowledging the costs and long-term consequences of living a sedentary lifestyle), determining personal goals (e.g., knowing what I want or need), and identifying the strategies needed to reach those goals (e.g., generating an action plan that replaces negative habits with positive routines). We turn now to an examples of applying the DVM to clients. First, a review of the model is warranted, followed by applying the model for two clients. See Anshel (2008, 2013) for a full description of the DVM.

Review of the DVM

The goal of this model is to strongly encourage a person to replace at least one unhealthy habits with one or more healthier routines. This is done by detecting an inconsistency between one or more of his or her most important values and actions. After acknowledging that the consequences of this inconsistency are not acceptable (for any one of several reasons), an action plan is generated jointly by the coach/therapist/health professional and the client that is intended to create at least one new, permanent habit. Let's briefly review each DVM component and then provide two sample applications.

Negative Habits

All of us have habits that may be categorized as "unhealthy" or not compatible with promoting energy and high-quality performance. We consciously experience these thoughts, emotions, and behaviors regularly, knowing they are unhealthy or not in our best interests, and yet remain under their control despite our ability to prevent or stop them. The result is low energy, premature mental and physical fatigue, excessive weight gain, and overall poor health, thereby compromising energy and quality of life.

Bad habits have benefits, without which people would not continue to exhibit them. The primary reason people engage in negative habits is because the perceived benefits of maintaining the habit outweigh its costs and long-term consequences. For example, the negative habit of failing to manage anger in response to frustration has the perceived "benefit" of prompting action by others, maintaining situational control, and the emotional release of unpleasant feelings. The "costs" of demonstrating acute anger (e.g., alienating others, poor social relationships, heightened stress) and long-term consequences (e.g., developing heart disease and hypertension, lack of respect and trust by others) are either not acknowledged or perceived as less important in meeting the person's short-term goals. Under these conditions, the negative habit persists.

Negative habits lead to performance barriers. Table 20.1 lists examples of negative/unhealthy habits for each of four dimensions of a healthy lifestyle: physical,

TABLE 20.1 Examples of Negative (Unhealthy) Habits that Lead to Performance Barriers

Physical	*Emotional*	*Mental/ Cognitive*	*Spiritual*
Lack of quality sleep	Poor communication skills	Self-critical; multitasker	Lack of passion about what really matters; low need to achieve
Sedentary lifestyle (lack of exercise)	Poor work/life balance	Inflexible	Lack of empathy
Poor hydration	Chokes under pressure	Defensive	Abuse of power; adult bully
High chronic stress	Rigid/inflexible	"Me first" attitude	Poor work/life balance
Excessive mental fatigue	Impatient	Short attention span	No goals or aspirations
Lacks proper assertiveness	Bully toward others	Poor coping skills	Lacks compassion; selfish; "me first" attitude
Persistent conflict	Poor organization	Sarcastic	Rarely gives praise
Excessive alcohol intake	No respect for others	Driven by guilt	Lacks proper values
Unkempt physical appearance	Lacks anger management skills	Driven by fear/ insecurity	Takes credit for the work of others
Low energy and fatigue	Poor decision-making skills	Chronic anxiety	Work lacks meaning and value
Poor nutrition	Poor time management	Mental fatigue	Lacks mentors or models
	Does not trust others	Poor concentration	Poor family relations

mental, emotional, and spiritual (values-based). Barriers can be actual (e.g., injury, anger, impatience) or perceived (e.g., time restraints, discomfort, mental fatigue, anxiety). They are almost always controllable and, thus, changeable. For instance, the emotional barrier of anxiety (i.e., worry) can be controlled by addressing the source(s) of concern (e.g., irrational and pessimistic thinking) and developing adaptation strategies (e.g., positive self-talk, self-analysis, distraction activities) that overcome these thoughts. Thus, persons who are uncomfortable and self-conscious about exercising in group settings and who are younger, fitter, and thinner can focus on their exercise regimen while ignoring others in the room. Individuals who have time restraints can develop time management strategies and obtain social support from significant others to allow for exercise time.

Perceived Benefits of Negative Habits

As indicated earlier, there are benefits to each of our negative (unhealthy) habits; it is often the "perceived" benefits of an unhealthy habit that compels people to continue. If there were no benefits to a negative habit, it would likely cease. Examples of so-called "benefits" of not exercising include more time to do other things, not experiencing the discomfort of physical exertion, additional expenses related to purchasing fitness club memberships and exercise clothing and shoes, and the mental discomfort that accompanies attending facilities inhabited with younger and fitter individuals. Possible *costs* to not exercising are perceived as less important than the benefits.

Costs and Long-Term Consequences of Negative Habits

It is well known that a sedentary lifestyle is accompanied by factors that compromise health, well-being, and quality of life, referred to in the model as "costs and long-term consequences."The costs include reduced fitness, weight gain, and higher stress and anxiety.The long-term consequences of these costs include poorer physical and mental health; reduced quality of life; and, in some cases, shorter lifespan.The important question that practitioners must ask their clients is "Are these costs acceptable?" If clients find these costs acceptable, then the negative habit of not exercising and maintaining a sedentary lifestyle will likely continue. If, however, the costs are far greater than the benefits, *and* the client concludes that these costs are *unacceptable*, then a change in behavior, that is, development of a new, healthier habit, is far more likely.

The process of behavior change is not complete yet, however. One factor still missing in the attempt to alter behavior permanently, or at least long term, is linking the costs and long-term consequences of the negative habit to the person's deepest values and beliefs.

Determining One's Deepest Values and Beliefs

Clients are given a written list of values—client beliefs about what is really important to them—and are either asked to rank them or are asked to write a check next to their top five values. One could speculate the typical designated values would include health, family, integrity, happiness, honesty, character, faith, excellence, commitment, and concern for others.

For instance, the decision to begin and maintain an exercise program is more likely if three processes occurred: (1) clients acknowledge that the costs and long-term consequences of a negative habit are greater than the benefits, (2) clients acknowledge that these costs run counter to the client's deepest values and beliefs about what is important, and (3) clients acknowledge that this discrepancy between the client's negative

TABLE 20.2 Personal Values Checklist (in alphabetical order)

Values List		*Top Five Ranked*
___ Beauty	___ Health	1.________
___ Character	___ Humility	2.________
___ Commitment	___ Humor	3.________
___ Compassion	___ Integrity	4.________
___ Concern for others	___ Kindness	5.________
___ Courage	___ Knowledge	
___ Creativity	___ Loyalty	
___ Excellence	___ Perseverance	
___ Fairness	___ Respect for others	
___ Faith	___ Responsibility	
___ Family	___ Security	
___ Freedom	___ Serenity	
___ Generosity	___ Service to others	
___ Genuineness	___ Wealth	
___ Happiness		

habits and at least one of his or her values is unacceptable. Thus, behavior change is more likely to be permanent when the client concludes that life satisfaction is linked to behaving in a way that is consistent with one's deepest values. Table 20.2 consists of a checklist of personal values from which clients are asked to rank their top five.

Establishing a Disconnect

To help clients detect an inconsistency between their values and their negative/unhealthy (self-destructive) habits, practitioners ask, "To what extent are your values consistent with your actions? If you value your health, for instance, do you have habits that are not good for you and, therefore, are inconsistent with your values? What about your family? Do you value your family? If you lead a sedentary lifestyle and are not involved in a program of exercise, yet one of your deepest values is to maintain good health, to what extent is your value inconsistent with your behavior? If you value friendship or loyalty, and yet you treat others disrespectfully or regularly demonstrate impatience or anger toward people who you want to become your friend, is there a 'disconnect' between your values (i.e., friendship, loyalty) and actions? Are the short-term costs and long-term consequences of these sample disconnects acceptable?"

Acceptability of the Disconnect

If clients acknowledge that the negative habit (e.g., not engaging in exercise, persistent anger or impatience) is inconsistent with their deepest values and beliefs about what is really important, these follow-up questions are needed: "Do you see a disconnect between your values (e.g., health, high quality of life, happiness) and any negative habits (e.g., lack of exercise, anger, impatience)? If a disconnect is acknowledged, is it acceptable, especially after identifying the costs and long-term consequences of this negative habit?"

Sometimes clients will feel that changing a negative habit is either undesirable, beyond their control, or can be "explained away." A "good" excuse can be articulated for the negative habit. In this situation, no change in behavior is likely to occur. I have observed many "reasons" for defending a person's current belief, attitude, emotion, or actions in which there is no wish to change. Health professionals have to find another disconnect between negative habits and values that clients feel are unacceptable. Clients are far more likely to commit to behavior change and to develop and carrying out an action plan if a designated disconnect is unacceptable, given the costs and consequences of maintaining the negative habit.

Developing an Action Plan

If the previous stages can be designated as "talking the talk," this stage can be called "walking the walk." This segment is about determining and initiating a plan to reduce or eliminate at least one negative habit and to replace it with a new, more desirable ritual that eliminates the disconnect between values and behaviors. The client's decision to initiate an exercise program, for instance, is ostensibly because the disconnect between the negative habit of nonexercise and his or her deepest values and beliefs is unacceptable. An action plan to prepare and carry out an exercise program follows.

The primary goal of the action plan consists of replacing the undesirable habit with a new, healthier one. For instance, the new habit of engaging in regular exercise includes knowing the type of exercise, exercise location(s), and days of the week and times of day to exercise; completion of a series of exercise tests to establish a baseline of fitness and other health indicators; and availability of social support (e.g., exercising with others, being held accountable for adhering to this new habit, determining the need for assistance by work mates, having family members support this new habit) and personal fitness coaching.

The results of past studies indicate that specificity of timing and precision of behavior dramatically increases the probability of successfully carrying out a self-controlled action plan. The action plan is similar to the actions of an elite athlete who engages in planning thoughts and actions before, during, and often immediately after executing the skill.

The action plan consists primarily of three factors that will markedly enhance the client's *permanent* commitment to regular exercise: (1) a specific time within a 24-hour period for exercise engagement; (2) a set of routines that support the exercise habit (e.g., selected thoughts and behaviors prior to, during, and following the exercise session, exercising with a friend and promoting other forms of social support, minimizing distractions that will interfere with exercise plans); and (3) linking these specific times and routines to the client's deepest values and beliefs about what is really important in life, resulting in removal of the existing disconnect.

Preliminary Information

Note: The present DVM program does not include a set of formal questions to ascertain personal information, background, and current habits, including the one or more the client wishes to change; it is suggested that the therapist/health care provider generate questions to help the session(s) focus on client needs and goals.

Case Study: Greg

Greg is a married, nonsmoking 52-year old male with one child. He stands 6 feet 2 inches tall, weighs 290 pounds, has 37% body fat (the average for males is 20–25%); and has a waist circumference of 51.5 inches. Greg's two main problems, perhaps not surprisingly, were the complete absence of regular (daily) exercise—he has a desk job and sits all day except for attending meetings and eating—and a high-fat, low-fiber diet. Greg is a former high school football athlete, so he is unsteady on his knees. He is unable to jog; aerobic exercise would have to be conducted either on a stationary bicycle or in the pool. As an athlete he lifted weights, so he is familiar with strength-training techniques and routines. His goals are to lose weight, increase muscular strength ("bulk up", as he put it), and to have more energy for his work and family.

Four people were involved in Greg's 10-week program, each of whom had a specific role in guiding him through the DVM. They were: (1) a licensed psychologist with a specialization in health-related issues (called a "life skills coach" to avoid any perceived stigma associated with obtaining professional counseling), (2) a registered dietician, (3) a personal trainer, and (4) a "performance coach" who was the central agent in guiding Greg through the DVM program. The performance coach was not credentialed to administer professional counseling but rather worked with the client to complete each stage of the DVM. The performance coach also referred the client to each of the other services, including a fitness coach based in a local exercise facility as well as a registered dietician and licensed therapist, both of whom practice near the home facility.

It is important to note that each of these involved professionals could have provided more than one role. For instance, each individual could have served as the performance coach as well as his or her respective area of expertise.

Before describing the role of each program coach, it is important to recognize that one of the most relevant features of being involved in the DVM program is more of an art than a science—the coach's communication skills, personality, and development of trust and credibility. Regardless of one's credentials and expertise, if the coach/specialist is unable to establish a warm and trusting relationship with his/her client, the coach will not have credibility, the client will not adopt program strategies, and the program will be ineffective. It is difficult, if not impossible, to teach personal skills. The coach must demonstrate sincerity in wanting to help make a difference in the client's life and to demonstrate genuineness and empathy in this journey toward enhancing quality of life. The client has to believe that each program-related person with whom he or she comes into contact sincerely wants to give that client 100% support and effort. Staff cannot fake their way through a program that is so personal and meaningful to each client. Clients can detect a "fake" coach almost immediately. Coach sincerity and integrity are required.

The role of each individual was concerned with the following issues:

Therapist. This person may be credentialed as a therapist, licensed professional counselor (LPC), social worker, or licensed psychologist (which requires a doctorate in psychology among many other requirements) and must serve an important function in the program. Their primary role was to provide insights into possible evidence of psychopathology, which may impede progress in the program and lead to dropping out (i.e., nonadherence to carrying out the action plan). It is important to indicate that this person was part of the support team in carrying out the program and did not constitute formal psychotherapy. He or she might detect the need for counseling and either refer the client to another therapist or agree to meet the client professionally as a separate component of the program in the therapist's professional office.

Sample topics that could require therapeutic intervention include dysfunctional eating patterns (e.g., emotional and passive eating), depression, low self-esteem, chronic anxiety, irrational thinking (e.g., "I don't deserve to be healthy"; "My husband/wife accepts me as obese"; "Past programs have not worked for me so why should this one?"), and other disorders.

Registered dietician. The registered dietician (RD) was responsible for the following tasks: (a) obtaining a copy of the client's lipids profile blood test and interpreting the blood test results; (b) reacting to the client's current eating habits and food intake; and (c) providing information about proper eating habits, called "strategic eating," that would promote high energy, weight loss, and improved lipid profile (blood test) scores. The RD helped clients make proper food choices that were sensitive to improper dietary preferences. In addition, the client (Greg) supplied a recent blood test that included a lipids profile of his cholesterol measures.

Fitness coach/personal trainer. The fitness coach/personal trainer—these titles are typically used interchangeably—should be employed at a local fitness club, university, or recreational program where certification and proper knowledge about improving fitness is usually required. There is an array of credentials and certification titles associated with knowledge and expertise in exercise and fitness. The key issue for certification concerns the person's ability to perform the following functions:

(a) provide a series of preprogram fitness tests (e.g., cardiovascular fitness, upper and lower body strength, percent body fat, blood pressure, waist circumference) to form a set of baseline scores against which to compare later test scores to detect improvement,

(b) provide clients with an exercise prescription that included resistance (weight) training and aerobic exercise to improve cardiovascular fitness, and

(c) measures of flexibility. All preprogram fitness tests would be repeated at the program's end, in this program, a period of 10 weeks. Although Greg was required to engage in three one-hour sessions of exercise per week, instruction was provided only one of the three hours per week. Greg was tested again at the end of the 10-week program (post-test) to ascertain improvement on the test scores.

The Orientation (allow for 90–120 minutes)

The first and primary step in applying the DVM, conducted by a separate performance coach or one of the specialty coaches, is the orientation. This segment includes six steps. See Appendix A for the DVM workbook that should be followed with the client.

1. First, Greg was to develop a mission statement about the intended outcomes of this 10-week program. After receiving instruction on creating mission statements, Greg was asked to identify the physical, mental, emotional, and spiritual reasons for improving his health and energy.
2. Second, in the model's cost-benefit tradeoff segment, Greg identified the negative habits that he felt most impaired his quality of life, energy, personal life (e.g., family, private time), and professional career. In order to understand the reasons he persisted at those undesirable habits, he listed their benefits. For example, the benefits of eating a fast food breakfast almost daily included good taste, low cost, convenience of the restaurant's location (i.e., on the way to his job), a feeling of fullness for much of the morning, and relatively good nutrition. Then he listed the "costs" of these habits, including high fat content, high number of ingested calories, higher expense than homemade breakfasts, and less nutrition than a properly prepared homemade breakfast. Long-term consequences were increased "bad" cholesterol, reduced "good" cholesterol, weight gain, and premature heart disease, even some cancers.
3. In the third segment, Greg was asked to identify *five* of his most important values. Greg listed family, faith, health, work quality/career, and character. Greg was then asked to make two lists, placed adjacent to each other.

   The list located on the left side of the page consisted of his unhealthy habits and performance barriers. The list included overeating; eating two meals a day from "fast food" restaurants; avoiding fresh vegetables and salads; not exercising; and eating pastry for dessert after lunch, as a midafternoon snack, and as a late night snack. The list located on the right side of the page consisted of a written list of his values, that is, issues about which he felt passionate.

4. He was then asked to compare the contents of each list and to identify and articulate aloud (to his performance coach—the program leader) any "disconnects," that is, areas in which a negative habit was inconsistent with a particular value. Four disconnects were located.

Greg was then asked to contemplate—with no set time limit—the following statement: "Given the costs and long-term consequences of at least one of your negative habits that is inconsistent with at least one of your deepest values, is this disconnect acceptable?"

He was informed that if he concluded the disconnect *was* acceptable, then he would maintain the negative habit; a change in his negative/unhealthy habit would likely persist. However, an *unacceptable disconnect* would indicate he acknowledges an inconsistency and that, given the costs and consequences of continuing this unhealthy habit, he would likely be ready to engage in an action plan to replace the negative habit (e.g., daily fast food breakfasts, lack of exercise) with positive, desirable routines. Greg agreed that his wife would fix a healthy breakfast at least three workdays per week—or he would fix breakfast himself—rather than eat the fast food restaurant's breakfast each day. Greg than met with each of the four coaches—RD, fitness, therapist (life skills coach), and performance coach—over the rest of the day to create new, healthier habits and remove the disconnects during the 10-week program.

Post-Test Results

All pretests were conducted again immediately after the program—called post-tests. Results indicated the following pretest and post-test comparisons.

(1) The lipids profile scores all improved (higher HDL, lower LDL, and triglycerides).
(2) Greg's weight was reduced from 290 to 282 pounds (it is important to note that Greg's one explanation of this relatively small decrease in body weight may be due to his increased musculature, as evident in his strength scores).
(3) There were significant improvements in upper- and lower-body strength based on the one-repetition strength test.
(4) Submaximal VO_2 score, a reflection if improved cardiovascular fitness, was improved (this test must be given by a certified fitness instructor).
(5) He blood pressure was reduced for both systole and diastole.
(6) His waistline circumference was reduced by three inches from 51.5 to 47 inches.
(7) His percent body fat was reduced from 37% to 33%.

Self-reporting—subjective data coming from the client—indicated increased perceived energy for work and family and a generally improved feeling of health and well-being.

Action Plan Adherence

Perhaps most significant was Greg's high rate of adherence to his exercise regimen. Full adherence was defined as attending exercise sessions a minimum of three times per week over the 10-week program, a total of 30 sessions. Greg attended 26 of the 30 sessions, or 87% adherence. A postprogram interview revealed that a combination of prayer and remembering to overcome his disconnected value system was imperative to maintaining his new set of routines related to eating behavior and exercise.

One-Time Action Steps

The primary focus of this program, which follows each stage of the DVM, is to motivate people to change certain aspects of their behavior—to get out of the comfort zone of unhealthy habits and to replace them with desirable, healthier routines. One factor that leads to maintaining behavior change, especially if the new behavior is uncomfortable or requires extra effort, is quick action, that is, to do something that will make an almost *immediate* impact. Intrinsic to this program is a strategy called "one-time action steps" that meets the needs of most individuals to adopt at least one activity that will make a very quick impact on one's health. People need to see rapid results, and one-time action steps help meet that need.

Table 20.3 lists sample one-time action steps from which clients can choose and adopt almost immediately after completing this program. It is imperative that this selection, even if adopting not more than one new action, be shared with the performance coach to improve accountability.

New Habits Adopted by Greg

Greg experienced a "reawakening" with respect to his lifestyle, poor health, and ignoring family, among other disconnected values. He adopted new rituals from the program that, over time, became healthy habits. Categorized by each dimension, they were as follows:

Physical habits: (a) started a new exercise program weekdays with a friend from work (on weekends with his wife); (b) ate breakfast at home (instead at the fast food restaurant each day), which reduced calories and increased fiber; (c) ate high-fiber snacks midmorning (fruit) and midafternoon (yogurt or an energy bar); (d) drank three bottles of water each day while at work; and (e) avoided anything stressful within two hours of bedtime.

TABLE 20.3 Sample One-Time Action Steps

Spiritual Capacity
Action Value (from values checklist) Date Started/Completed
Find a mentor
Become a mentor
Join a spiritual center or organization
Donate money or time to charity
Pray
Spend more time with family
Others:
Emotional Capacity
Buy a gift or send a card to someone special
Adopt a pet
Communication frequently/regularly with partner/family members
Plan and take a trip/vacation with partner/significant other
Perform community service
Start a new hobby
Phone someone special
Others:
Mental Capacity
Purchase a calendar/appointment book
Manage time to allow for recovery periods during the day
Buy a new book
Start a new magazine/journal/newspaper subscription
Register for a new course
Take regular recovery breaks during the day
Insert new (positive) rituals into daily routines
Others:
Physical Capacity
Eat breakfast
Join a fitness club
Hire a personal trainer
Schedule a massage
Buy a heart rate monitor
Have a stress test
Register for a yoga course
Purchase new fitness clothing/equipment
Other:

Mental habits: Greg's exercise routine and improved sleep seemed to translate into superior concentration at work, being more attentive to his family members during conversations, and displaying more rational (less work addiction and perfectionism) and more accurate work-related decision making. An additional mental habit Greg learned was to improve his coping skills following stressful events. Greg's reaction to stressful situations was usually nonconstructive and actually increased his stress level. If work-related, he usually brought stressful feelings home with him. His new habit, however, was to leave sources of stress at work and to schedule enjoyable events at home in the evenings. He learned "avoidance coping" in which he was able to psychologically distance himself from the source of stress and not take everything so seriously.

Emotional habits: Greg dealt with his moodiness—especially upon arriving to work in the early morning—by adopting a technique called "Act as if. . ." This technique consists of generating a script that places the person in a professional and friendly mindset upon entering the workplace. Greg "acted as if" he was in a positive frame of mind, greeting colleagues with "good morning" and a smile; if he was genuinely curious about an issue, he would address it at that time. Comments were always upbeat, complimentary, and sincere. He patiently waited for his colleague's reply and replied to the comment before commenting or going to the next issue. Greg also adopted new nonverbal skills, such as looking at colleagues in the eye when speaking to them and showing interest in their words by nodding as they spoke. This set of communication strategies built trust, loyalty, respect, and genuineness within the company.

Spiritual habits: Greg has a strong spiritual side to his life, but it was expressed negatively. He felt little passion toward his work due to stress and putting far too much time into work demands. He also had the bad habit of ignoring his family and coming home well past dinner time, although he ate dinner at home most nights.

He set aside time with his family, especially spending alone time with his son. He also adopted a strategy called "date night" in which he went out for dinner at least one time per week and, sometimes, a movie or other entertainment with his wife. Another spiritual issue was to recognize the disconnects between his values—family, health, work performance, faith—and his actions. Greg felt that he needed to reconnect with his place of worship and attended weekly services with his family. He also needed to remove the disconnects between his values and unhealthy or undesirable habits, and this decision literally changed his quality of life.

One-time action steps: One-time strategies included purchasing a book on exercise strategies to improve cardiovascular fitness. In addition, he hired a personal trainer who conducted three fitness tests to establish baseline scores, and he gave his wife a fitness club membership for their anniversary under the condition that they exercise together at least one time per week at the club.

Implications for Practitioners and Future Directions

The DVM is intended to serve as an intervention tool for therapists, coaches, medical and mental health practitioners, religious leaders, and consultants, with or without a credential or license to practice counseling. We live in a culture that promotes unhealthy habits and are surrounded by others—family, work colleagues, personal friends—who accept our way of life and the medical problems that come with the way we live (e.g., "My whole family is overweight; I can't help it"). The conditions that lead to poor health, obesity, low energy, and low life satisfaction are often self-imposed. Some individuals refuse to take personal responsibility for their actions—low self-control—and attribute their poor health and other undesirable characteristics to factors outside their control such as genetics, a "higher power," fate, or cultural food habits. It is imperative to help clients take more personal responsibility for their actions that lead to unhealthy, self-destructive outcomes.

How do you help others change habits? This is the key question in administering any behavior change intervention, including the DVM. The DVM consists primarily of replacing one set of behaviors, deemed "negative" or unhealthy, with another set of behaviors, labeled positive or healthy. The DVM does not include psychotherapy and other skills that require licensure as a psychologist (although possessing the licensure credential is not a disadvantage), thus allowing practitioners with an array of skills and interests to apply the model in various settings.

For optimal effectiveness in applying the DVM, it is important that the practitioner have the following: (1) possess superb communication skills, including empathy, genuineness, and warmth; (2) establish a close, trusting relationship with the client; (3) engage with the client in a quiet, isolated environment to promote privacy and confidentiality; (4) promise strict confidentiality about information the client provides; (5) avoid judging the client's feelings and actions; (6) provide support to carry out the action plan (e.g., establishing partners, identifying needed equipment or resources, suggest programs or partners); and (7) monitor progress with follow-up sessions to ensure adherence.

Another important implication for practitioners in applying the DVM intervention concerns assessing the client's behaviors. Was the intervention efficacious? Did the client establish new rituals that were intended to improve health and establish a consistency with his or her values? Did the client remove the disconnect between his or her values and unhealthy habits? Assessing the model's efficacy requires behavioral assessment.

Examples of behavioral assessment include interviewing (e.g., identifying negative habits such as not exercising), behavioral inventories (e.g., determining selected psychological dispositions that are associated with inactivity), task-relevant behavioral checklists (e.g., self-monitoring that provides instructional feedback on proper exercise skills or executing an effective fitness program), and performance profiling (e.g., asking clients to self-examine their attitudes, perceived barriers, level of mastery, and other factors that might promote or impede future exercise participation).

Finally, as Glasgow et al. (2004) have concluded about the future of health behavior change research, "If we are serious about evidence-based behavioral medicine and about closing the gap between research findings and application of these findings in applied settings, we cannot continue 'business as usual'" (p. 11).

New, creative approaches to changing health behavior are needed. Getting rid of one (self-destructive) habit and replacing it with another (superior) one remains a major challenge in health care that requires full psychological and physical client readiness to examine one's current status with regard to health, happiness, and quality of life. There is no magic bullet.

References

Anshel, M. H. (2008). The Disconnected Values Model: Intervention strategies for health behavior change. *Journal of Clinical Sport Psychology, 2*, 357–380.

Anshel, M. H. (2013). A cognitive-behavioral approach for promoting exercise behavior: The Disconnected Values Model. *Journal of Sport Behavior, 36*, 107–129.

Glasgow, R.E., Klesges, L.M., Dzewaltowski, D. A., Bull, S.S., & Estabrooks, P. (2004). The future of health behavior change research: What is needed to improve translation of research into health promotion practice. *Annals of Behavioral Medicine, 27*, 3–12.

Hogan, H.W., & Mookherjee, H.N. (1981). Values and selected antecedents. *Journal of Social Psychology, 113*, 29–35.

Rokeach, M. (1973). *The nature of human values*. New York: Free Press.

Super, D.E. (1995). Values: Their nature, assessment, and practical use. In D. E. Super & B. Sverko (Eds.), *Life roles, values, and careers: International findings of the work importance study* (pp. 54–61). San Francisco: Jossey-Bass.

ADDITIONAL READINGS

Anshel, M.H. (2006). *Applied exercise psychology: A practitioner's guide to improving client health and fitness*. New York: Springer Publishing Company.

Anshel, M.H., & Brinthaupt, T.M. (2012). Enhancing community and campus wellness: Application of the Disconnected Values Model. In A. M. Columbus (Ed.), *Advances in psychology research* (Vol. 90, pp. 41–64). Hauppauge, NY: Nova Science Publishers.

Anshel, M.H., & Kang, M. (2007). Effect of an intervention on replacing negative habits with Positive routines for improving full engagement at work: A test of the Disconnected Values Model. *Journal of Consulting Psychology: Practice and Research, 59*, 110–125.

Anshel, M.H., & Kang, M. (2007). An outcome-based action study on changes in fitness, blood lipids, and exercise adherence based on the Disconnected Values Model. *Behavioral Medicine, 33*, 85–98.

Anshel, M.H. (2008). The Disconnected Values Model: Intervention strategies for health behavior change. *Journal of Clinical Sport Psychology, 2*, 357–380.

Anshel, M.H., & Kang, M. (2008). Effectiveness of motivational interviewing on changes in fitness, blood lipids, and exercise adherence among police officers. *Journal of Correctional Health Care, 14*, 48–62.

Anshel, M. H. (2010). The Disconnected Values (Intervention) Model for promoting health habits in religious institutions. *Journal of Religion and Health, 49*, 32–49.

Anshel, M. H. (2013). A cognitive-behavioral approach for promoting exercise behavior: The Disconnected Values Model. *Journal of Sport Behavior, 36*, 107–129.

Anshel, M.H. (2014). *Applied health fitness psychology*. Champaign, IL: Human Kinetics.

Anshel, M. H., Kang, M., & Brinthaupt, T. M. (2010). Promoting health behavior change with the Disconnected Values Model: An action study. *International Journal of Sport and Exercise Psychology, 8*, 413–433.

Baranowski, T., Anderson, C., & Carmack, C. (1998). Mediating variable framework in physical activity interventions. How are we doing? How might we do better? *American Journal of Preventive Medicine, 15*, 266–297.

Brinthaupt, T. M., Kang, M., & Anshel, M. H. (2010). A delivery model for overcoming psycho- behavioral barriers to exercise. *Psychology of Sport & Exercise, 11*, 259–266.

Brinthaupt, T. M., Kang, M., & Anshel, M. H. (2013). Changes in exercise commitment following a values-based wellness program. *Journal of Sport Behavior, 36*, 3–22.

Goldstein, A.P. *Reducing resistance: Methods for enhancing openness to change*. Champaign, IL: Research Press.

Lox, C.L., Martin, K.A., & Petruzzello, S.J. (2014). *The psychology of exercise: Integrating theory and practice* (4th ed.). Scottsdale, AZ: Holcomb Hathaway.

Marcus, B.H., & Forsythe, L.H. (2003). *Motivating people to be physically active*. Champaign, IL: Human Kinetics.

Marcus, B.H., King, T.K., Bock, B. C., Borrelli, B., & Clark, M.M. (1998). Adherence to physical activity recommendations and interventions. In S. A. Shumaker, E. B. Schron, J. K. Ockene, & W. L. McBee (Eds.), *The handbook of health behavior change* (2nd ed., 189–212). New York: Springer.

Schumaker, S.A., Ockene, J.K., & Riekert, K.A. (Eds., 2009). *The handbook of health behavior change* (3rd ed.). New York: Springer Publishing Company.

APPENDIX A

Sample Client Workbook for Applying the Disconnected Values Model

DVM book users, this section contains a handout to clients—individuals and groups—when applying the DVM. While you may use some or all of this material, it's important that each stage be fully carried out so that participants are properly motivated with a sense of purpose in making health-related changes and begin the process of linking their values to living a healthy lifestyle. Be sure you have a supply of pens/pencils to distribute to participants so they go through the process together and record their responses for immediate and future use.

The Disconnected Values Model: Cognitive-Behavioral Intervention Strategies for Replacing Unhealthy Habits, Thoughts, Emotions, and Behavior Patterns

Intervention leader's name and contact information here:

Presentation Objectives

(1) To examine the impediments and barriers to health behavior change—why our culture engages in self-destructive behavior patterns;
(2) To help clients acknowledge the benefits and costs of their negative habits;
(3) To experience stages of the Disconnected Values Model that posit that our "bad" behavior patterns are inconsistent with—"disconnected" from—our values; and
(4) To generate and carry out an action plan in which unhealthy habits are replaced by more desirable routines in an attempt to live a life consistent with our deepest values and beliefs, promote health and energy, and improve quality of life.

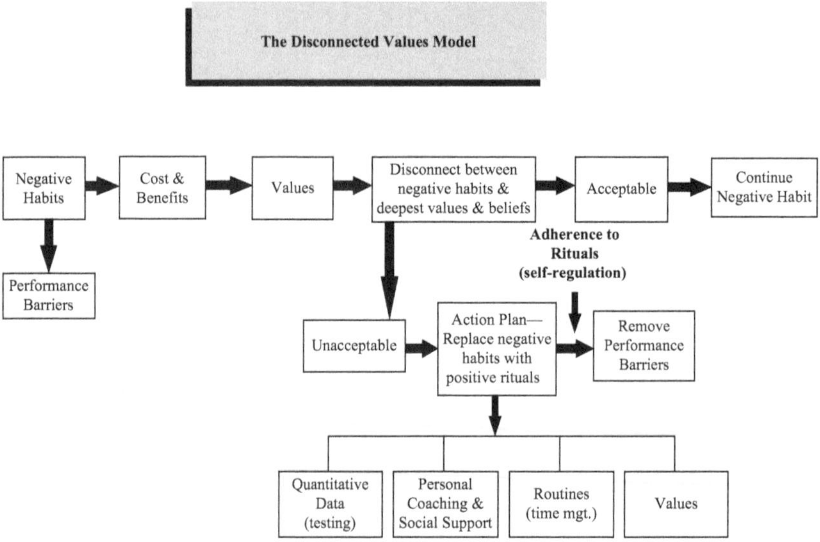

Common reasons for unhealthy, self-destructive behaviors: (1) Benefits of unhealthy habits are immediate, whereas costs and consequences are long term, often many years away; and (2) benefits outweigh the costs and consequences. We have a culture based on immediate gratification, not a culture that thrives on the benefits of delayed gratification.

Confronting the Cost and Benefit Tradeoff

	Client's Current Bad Habit	*Benefit of Current Bad Habit*	*Cost of Bad Habit*	*Long-Term Consequences of Bad Habit*
1				
2				
3				
4				
5				
6				

	Client's Current Bad Habit	*Benefit of Current Bad Habit*	*Cost of Bad Habit*	*Long-Term Consequences of Bad Habit*
	Sample Content			
7	**Poor Diet (high fat, high sugar)**	**Immediate gratification; convenience, low cost**	**High cholesterol; increased weight; less sustained positive energy**	**Increased risk of obesity, heart disease, strokes, cancer, and early death**
8	**Anger, impatience, bullying, and defensiveness toward others**	**Keeps people at a safe distance; avoids responsibility; maintains control**	**Alienates coworkers; undermines teamwork; negative mood**	**Isolation; rigidity; poor relationships; failure to grow and improve quality of work; leads to burnout.**
9	**Excessive alcohol and drug abuse**	**Immediate pleasure; reduced tension and anxiety; greater social ease**	**Impaired concentration; erratic work performance; mood swings; troubled relationships**	**Higher health risks; undermines relationships, self-esteem, and performance**
10	**No Exercise**	**More time for work and other obligations; less effort**	**Less energy, strength, general well-being; lost source of recovery from mental activities; more susceptibility to sickness**	**Undermines health; lowers concentration and access to high positive energy; increases chances of early death**

Common Barriers that Compromise Health, Energy, and Performance

Circle **five** of the most important/destructive barriers that affect your life.

1. Lack of assertiveness and self-direction
2. Poor team player (thinks "me" not "we")
3. Constant conflict with boss or coworker

4. Poor fitness
5. Poor organization and time management
6. Low motivation and passion at work
7. Fear and insecurity on the job
8. Poor communication skills
9. Low stress tolerance
10. Rigid and inflexible
11. Poor sleep habits
12. Low energy and fatigue
13. Poor work/life balance
14. Poor nutrition and hydration
15. Lack of trust in others
16. Lack of discipline and follow through
17. Lack of empathy and compassion
18. Negative and pessimistic thinker
19. Impatience, frustration, and anger
20. Failure to connect work to deepest values and beliefs
21. Poor relationships in personal life
22. Low control over own actions
23. Short attention span

Values Checklist: Check three of your most important values

Balance	❐	Happiness	❐
Beauty	❐	Harmony	❐
Character	❐	Health	❐
Commitment	❐	Humor	❐
Commitment	❐	Humility	❐
Concern for others	❐	Integrity	❐
Courage	❐	Kindness	❐
Creativity	❐	Knowledge	❐
Excellence	❐	Loyalty	❐
Faith	❐	Perseverance	❐
Fairness	❐	Respect for others	❐
Family	❐	Responsibility	❐
Freedom	❐	Security	❐
Generosity	❐	Serenity	❐
Genuineness	❐	Service to others	❐
		Wealth	❐

Find at least one disconnect (inconsistency) between your barriers and values. Given the costs and long-term consequences of this disconnect, is this disconnect acceptable?

Important Rituals to Expand Physical Capacity

Nutrition and Hydration

1. Eat three meals and two snacks daily.
2. Eat breakfast daily.
3. Never go longer than four hours without food.
4. Eat 40% grains, 40% fruits and vegetables, and 20% protein.
5. Eat no more than five handfuls of food per meal (portion control).
6. Snacks should be 100 to 150 calories; include fruit. Snacking is a healthy habit.
7. 80% of one's food intake at any meal should be from *need* foods and 20% from *want* foods.
8. Eat until you are satisfied, not full.
9. Drink water regularly throughout the day, preferably 64 oz. or more.
10. Alcohol, if consumed, should be with meals. Two glasses/day maximum.
11. Keep caffeinated beverages to a minimum; do not consume caffeine within two hours of bedtime.

Exercise/Physical Activity

1. Every 30 to 45 minutes, perform small movements.
2. Every 90 to 120 minutes, perform major movements.
3. Go to bed early and wake up early.
4. Do some form of physical activity daily.
5. Do at least two strength training workouts per week.
6. Do at least two cardiovascular interval workouts per week.
7. To expand capacity, expend energy to the feeling of discomfort.
8. Breathe from the diaphragm to enhance energy recovery.
9. Exercise at moderate to high intensity to improve cardiovascular capacity and burn more calories.
10. Ideal exercise length is 30–60 minutes, 3–5 times per week.
11. TAKE STEPS; avoid prolonged sitting. Walk around or do something physical at least every 90 min.

Sleep/Presleep Rituals

1. Go to bed and wake up consistently at the same times.
2. Sleep is usually higher quality earlier at night; "early to bed, early to rise."
3. Get seven to eight hours of sleep each night. Highly fit individuals may require less.
4. Avoid full meals within two hours of bedtime.
5. Avoid caffeine and alcohol within two hours of bedtime (they are diuretics, which increase arousal and urinary output, disturbing sleep).
6. Avoid stress within two hours of bedtime.

7. Beware of sleep apnea (cessation of breathing during sleep); predicts stroke and heart attack.
8. Do something relaxing that reduces intense or unpleasant feelings, even going for a walk. Be sure there is a gap of time between computer use and bedtime.
9. Avoid watching television in your bedroom (according to the National Sleep Foundation).

Twenty-Four-Hour Time Management Worksheet

Value	Sample Value: Health	**New Ritual**	Daily brisk walking/resistance training
Value	Sample Value: Family	**New Ritual**	Get proper rest to maintain energy for family. Spend more time with kids.
Value		**New Ritual**	
Value		**New Ritual**	

4:00 a.m.	4:00 p.m.
4:30 a.m.	4:30 p.m.
5:00 a.m.	5:00 p.m.
5:30 a.m.	5:30 p.m.
6:00 a.m.	6:00 p.m.
6:30 a.m.	6:30 p.m.
7:00 a.m.	7:00 p.m.
7:30 a.m.	7:30 p.m.
8:00 a.m.	8:00 p.m.
8:30 a.m.	8:30 p.m.
9:00 a.m.	9:00 p.m.
9:30 a.m.	9:30 p.m.
10:00 a.m.	10:00 p.m.
10:30 a.m.	10:30 p.m.
11:00 a.m.	11:00 p.m.
11:30 a.m.	11:30 p.m.
Noon	Midnight
12:30 p.m.	12:30 a.m.
1:00 p.m.	1:00 a.m.
1:30 p.m.	1:30 a.m.
2:00 p.m.	2:00 a.m.
2:30 p.m.	2:30 a.m.
3:00 p.m.	3:00 a.m.
3:30 p.m.	3:30 a.m.

Required inserted activities: meals, snacks, sleep, waking up, exercise, recovery breaks, reflection, and planning time.

Mental Skills for Exercise

Your thoughts really do influence emotions, mood, effort, and exercise performance. Here are suggestions taken from the exercise psychology literature that help promote exercise performance and outcomes. I divided these mental skills into two components, pre-exercise skills and exercise-related skills.

I. Pre-Exercise *Mental Skills*

1. Develop an exercise routine; schedule it. Ultimately, the goal of any exerciser is to ritualize his or her fitness program. Researchers claim that we thrive on rituals because they help reduce stress, cut down on the number of things we have to plan and think about, and promote overall well-being. An exercise ritual—scheduling our exercise times and locations—reduces the chance of "forgetting" or running out of time to exercise.

2. Receive proper instruction and coaching. Exercise is a science; there is a right way and a wrong way to perform it. Listen to your coach and ask questions.

3. Develop a positive attitude and self-confidence toward exercise. The enthusiasm you feel toward any task or program will result in better adherence and superior outcomes. See the "big picture" about the benefits—short term and long term—of your involvement, and be committed to experience the full program. Do not let others or one or two individual experiences control your destiny. This is your health and quality of life we are talking about. Feel confident in your ability to learn and improve, and expect to receive all the benefits you deserve from the energy you are investing in this program. Along these lines, remember to live a life that is consistent with your values (e.g., health, family, high-quality job performance, faith, excellence, and so on).

4. Have realistic but challenging performance (not outcome) goals. The extensive research on goal setting is clear; goals tend to increase motivation, help the performer focus his or her energy toward the desired outcome, and fulfill a personal need to achieve and to feel competent, both of which are normal and desirable. To have goals that are credible, however, be sure your goals are challenging but realistic. Although a few beginning exercisers decide to train for eventually running a marathon (i.e., a 26-mile race) this is not realistic thinking for most of us.

5. Obtain fitness tests. Humans thrive on data—numbers from test results—that motivate us to change behavior. Ask any doctor about the best motivator to change their patients' unhealthy habits. Fitness testing also provides your coach with direction to provide an accurate exercise prescription.

6. Positive Pre-Exercise Thoughts. Have you ever said to yourself, before attending a fitness facility or before exercising, "I don't want to do this" or "Do I really have to exercise today?" What about the content of your thoughts during exercise? Positive (e.g., "I can do this"; "I feel good") or negative (e.g., "I am not enjoying this"; "This really sucks")? Studies show that the content of your thinking—positive or negative—can influence your mood, attitude, and energy level.

II. Exercise-Related *Mental Skills*

1. Positive self-talk: Although discussed earlier, this is a strategy that is essential to good exercise performance. Before your exercise session, be optimistic about the likely outcomes of your exercise session and of your involvement in the program, and—equally important—think "upbeat" thoughts *during* your exercise session. Your energy level, and hence, exercise performance, will actually improve in response to positive self-talk, as opposed to thinking negative thoughts.

2. Association: Association refers to connecting one's thoughts to bodily sensations, that is, focusing on specific body parts and muscle groups during exertion. Thus, when lifting weights, the exerciser uses association by focusing his or her attention on the muscles most heavily involved in that lift. When performing a bicep curl, for example, exercisers would focus their attention on the bicep muscle primarily responsible for that action. In response to cardiovascular activity, runners use association to think about the bodily sensations during the run—connecting thoughts to actions. Less fit folks prefer to *not use* association during cardiovascular exercise because those thoughts are not always pleasant. Instead, they would use dissociation.

3. Dissociation: Instead of focusing on the muscles being used or the bodily sensations being experienced during exercise, dissociation is concerned with disconnecting one's mind with one's exertion. The use of music when performing physical activity, especially when exercise is performed in synchronization to music, is a good example of a dissociation strategy. The person is focusing his or her attention on external stimuli rather than on bodily sensations experienced during exercise. Dissociation is a common technique used during cardiovascular work but not weight training, in which your attentional focus should be on the muscle group being exerted.

4. Bizarre imagery: This strategy concerns thinking about the impossible. Imagery concerns visualizing an action, that is, a mental representation of performance. Bizarre imagery means that the thought content cannot occur in reality yet is motivational to the performer. Examples include thinking about "washing away" plaque against the walls of arteries or having your fat "melt away" when performing aerobic activity. Cancer patients have used bizarre imagery to image shrinking tumors when receiving chemotherapy.

5. Music: Have you ever participated in an aerobics class in which you were moving to music—and felt more energy than when exercising in the absence of music? Music is a distractor, helping the person focus on external (musical) stimuli while the person gives minimal attention to bodily sensations associated with physical effort (e.g., fatigue, sweating, exertion, high heart rate, discomfort).

Exercising with fast-paced music tends to increase arousal level, which allows the person to move with greater intensity. Slower-paced music reduces arousal and heart rate; relaxation increases.

6. Social support: If you like to exercise with a friend or receive recognition from friends, family, or colleagues, you are experiencing social support. Social support is one of the leading predictors of exercise adherence. Social support can be direct (e.g., exercising with another person or receiving instruction or coaching) or indirect (e.g., others offer praise, recognition, or approval without exercising with you). Some individuals, however, prefer to exercise alone or do not find it motivating to receive attention from others.

7. Psyching up: The goal here is to improve arousal level, excitation, or positive emotion, which, in turn, increases effort and physical exertion. Examples of psyching-up strategies can be verbal (e.g., "Come on, I can do this"; "Go for it"; "Let's get this done"; "Do it, do it, do it") or nonverbal (e.g., increasing exertion during a particular phase of an exercise, perhaps when lifting weights).

In summary, mental skills are often ignored or not known to exercisers yet have an important role in improving exercise performance. There is a strong link between the mind and body, and what you think (also called cognition) and feel (emotion) will directly influence your physical performance. Many of these strategies are used by world-class athletes as part of their training and during competition.

Review of Main Concepts of This Program

Here is a review of the most important concepts that were part of this program.

1. *Changing health behavior*: The main components of any health behavior change model consist of developing new routines that are scheduled (i.e., days of the week, time of day) and are strongly supported by your deepest values and beliefs (i.e., feeling passionate about what is really important in your life).

2. *Goal of the DVM*: To replace negative, unhealthy habits with positive, healthier routines (that usually takes six to eight weeks).

3. *Expanding capacity*: The program addresses four dimensions that we want to go from *limited* to *expanded*. That is, we want to expand your capacity to have more energy, to perform at optimal levels, and to improve your quality of life.

a. Expanding your ***physical capacity*** is comprised of improving your energy due to (1) *exercise*, (2) improved *nutrition*, (3) *better hydration*, and (4) adequate *sleep*. Limitations in any of these will limit your capacity to perform optimally.
b. Expanding ***emotional capacity*** entails improved *self-awareness* about what we do, often daily, that compromises our health and well-being; improving our sense of *self-control* over our actions, thoughts, and emotions. Examples include: Do I *really* need that piece of cake or ice cream before bedtime? Can I replace pastry with fruit, yogurt, or cottage cheese, at least occasionally?

Should I care what others think when I exercise? Should I show *compassion and empathy* toward others and demonstrate competent *social skills*?

c. Expanding ***mental capacity*** means the ability to use effective time management so we act in ways that help us reach our goals (including time for exercise), to process information efficiently, to improve and maintain our concentration, and to adapt to the internal and external "storms" of life—a process called "values-based" adaptation, rather than "expedient" adaptation, the latter meaning short-term benefits but long-term negative consequences.

d. Finally, expanding ***spiritual capacity*** is about acknowledging your values (i.e., what you feel passionate about, what moves you) and leading a life that is consistent with those values. For example, if one of your values is *family*, yet you do not look after your health (e.g., no exercise, poor eating habits), there is a disconnect between your values and your actions. Expanding spiritual capacity is the ability to acknowledge this disconnect and then replace unhealthy habits with routines that bring your life into realignment with your values.

4. Cost-benefit tradeoff: There are benefits to every unhealthy (negative) habit or we would not continue to do them. What we rarely think about, however, are the costs and long-term consequences of these negative habits. Yes, we can use our power to intimidate others but at what cost to our relationships; our need for loyalty; and the wonderful feelings we derive from helping others learn, improve, and succeed? There are benefits to not exercising, eating high-fat food, and leading a life that is void of balance (e.g., all work, no time for family or, conversely, abusing the privilege of tenure and not giving 100% to your job).

Here's the key question: Given the costs and long-term consequences of your negative habits, is the disconnect between your values and unhealthy habits **acceptable?** If it is acceptable, then your negative habit will continue. No behavior change (after all, you're not dead—yet). However, if you conclude that this disconnect is **unacceptable,** due to the eventual consequences of the unhealthy habit/s, than you are ready to engage in an *action plan* that will replace the unhealthy habit with positive routines that will improve energy and quality of life.

5. Disconnects: Remember the two pages we completed during the orientation? They were "Most Common Barriers. . ." and the "Values Checklist." Reexamine the disconnects you identified. Hopefully, you will conclude that at least one (or more) of the disconnects you identified is acceptable, given the costs and consequences of maintaining it. One more thing: There are others, your family is first, then your work colleagues and students, who are depending on you to be available and accessible, to remain healthy so they can share their life with you, and for you to create a lasting and proud legacy—both at home and work. Realigning your daily habits with your values is only partly about you; it's also about the people you leave behind when you retire or die. Strong stuff, I know, but we need to think about what it will take to be happy and how we want to be remembered.

6. Act as if. . .: Our actions dictate our physiology and are more important than our thoughts. If, for example, you jumped up and down while yelling "I'm miserable," "I'm miserable," you'd likely laugh and feel positive. This is because the jumping action is more powerful than words or thoughts. Therefore, act "as if" you feel good; you are energized; and you are performing in the high, positive energy cell (Ideal Performance State). When you walk through the door at work, you are "on." No one needs to know you did not sleep well (no one cares, anyway). Act upbeat and professional. Keep up a positive frame of mind and *act as if* you are in a positive mood state. You WILL feel better as a result.

7. Action Plan and One-Time Action Steps: The program ends with an *action plan*, which consists of a time-managed schedule of events that, when integrated into your daily routine, becomes a positive habit. *One-time action steps* consist of a single decision and follow-up action that initiates the health behavior change process and expands your capacity to overcome barriers and reach desirable goals.

Remember this program's motto: **NEVER SURRENDER!** You are on a journey that will change the way you live, work, relate, and think. Please take your efforts at behavior change—as difficult and challenging as it is to change habits—very seriously. Time to celebrate the future.

APPENDIX B

Exerciser Checklist: Guidelines for High Quality Exercise Experiences

Applying the Exercise Checklist

Health consultants, coaches, and therapists can use a checklist in various ways to ensure that clients will adopt its content. Checklists can be developed for helping clients acquire any new habit or ritual. This is an exercise example. Here are some guidelines for generating and using checklists:

(1) *A checklist should be very focused in its goal(s) and purpose.* Is it strictly an information tool? Does it provide insights into proper exercise preparation and execution? Is it about developing healthy lifestyle habits? Does it address a particular type of exercise or address the needs of a special group or population?

(2) *Keep the checklist relatively brief and clear to the intended audience.* Users should be able to go through the checklist quickly; it should provide a very complete list of tasks that need to be done in order to experience a successful exercise session.

(3) *Begin your checklist with instructions that are brief and easy to comprehend.*

(4) *Keep the scoring consistent for all items.* For easy use, circling a "1" should always represent a low, undesirable score, while "5" reflects a score that is high and desirable. That is, clients should be able to add up their scores and conclude that achieving a higher score represents improvement or achievement over time.

(5) *Can it be easily read*? Similar to validating an inventory for research purposes, be sure that intended users understand the instructions for each item. Give the checklist a "trial run" by having several clients read it through and indicate if there are any words with which they are unfamiliar, if they are unsure about how to complete the checklist, or if they do not know what they must do to improve their score.

(6) *Allow for individual differences.* Some items may not even pertain to them. For instance, some individuals prefer to exercise alone, and clients should not feel compelled to exercise with others (if that was a checklist item). Items that are not relevant to a particular client should be deleted for that individual, rather than self-reporting a low score.

(7) *Provide live support for using the checklist.* Health care professionals, fitness coaches, dieticians, or anyone else associated with generating and using the checklist should work with the client in reviewing each response and how to improve item scores. Then, the client and staff member should agree to meet and carry out certain segments of the checklist to help improve item scores.

(8) *Provide clients with positive feedback.* Inform clients with messages of improvement and effort in carrying out the checklist content. It is essential that clients feel they are achieving goals toward improved health and fitness.

Listed below is an exercise self-monitoring checklist that can be generated to fit the needs of each client and would guide the client to engage in a high-quality fitness program. Please indicate how much you agree or disagree with each of the following statements concerning your exercise routine. The ratings go from **1** (the statement is not at all like me) to **5** (the statement is very much like me). Higher scores are viewed as more desirable than lower scores. You want to improve your score over time.

1	2	3	4	5
Not at All Like Me		**Somewhat Like Me**		**Very Much Like Me**

I. Exercise Preparation					
1. I think about exercising with enthusiasm.	1	2	3	4	5
2. I look forward to the next exercise session.	1	2	3	4	5
3. I do not make excuses for avoiding exercise.	1	2	3	4	5
4. I view exercising as a challenge, not a chore.	1	2	3	4	5
5. I feel healthier and happier for exercising.	1	2	3	4	5
6. I make time for exercise.	1	2	3	4	5
7. I am confident with my exercise technique.	1	2	3	4	5
8. My family/friends support my exercise habit.	1	2	3	4	5
9. I have a weekly exercise schedule.	1	2	3	4	5
10. I know the physical and psychological benefits of exercising regularly.	1	2	3	4	5
11. I would describe my lifestyle during the week as physically active.	1	2	3	4	5
12. I feel comfortable exercising alone or in the presence of others.	1	2	3	4	5

Subtotal: ______

1	2	3	4	5
Not at All Like Me		**Somewhat Like Me**		**Very Much Like Me**

II. Day of Exercise

1. I look forward to exercising with great enthusiasm.	1	2	3	4	5
2. I am committed to my scheduled exercise time.	1	2	3	4	5
3. I have prepared a proper diet and fluid intake today.	1	2	3	4	5
4. I am feeling positive about exercising.	1	2	3	4	5
5. I am aware of the benefits of my exercise program.	1	2	3	4	5
6. Within two hours of exercising, I will not have any intake of food, coffee, or alcohol.	1	2	3	4	5
7. If I feel sick, I will not exercise today.	1	2	3	4	5
8. I have a planned route to the exercise venue.	1	2	3	4	5
9. I have prepared my exercise gear in advance.	1	2	3	4	5
10. I have organized my day to accommodate my exercise session.	1	2	3	4	5

Subtotal: ______

1	2	3	4	5
Not at All Like Me		**Somewhat Like Me**		**Very Much Like Me**

III. Pre-Exercise Activity (at exercise venue)

1. I arrive at the exercise venue on time/with enthusiasm.	1	2	3	4	5
2. I remember my goals and plan to meet them.	1	2	3	4	5
3. As I prepare to exercise, I feel energetic.	1	2	3	4	5
4. I plan to have adequate water intake when I exercise.	1	2	3	4	5
5. I have an exercise plan.	1	2	3	4	5
6. I remember the reasons that exercise is good for me.	1	2	3	4	5
7. I will do as much of the exercise session as I can.	1	2	3	4	5
8. I use positive self-talk just before I exercise ("I can do it"; "I'm ready"; "Stay with it!")	1	2	3	4	5

1	2	3	4	5
Not at All Like Me		**Somewhat Like Me**		**Very Much Like Me**

IV. During My Exercise Session

1. I really enjoyed my exercise session.	1	2	3	4	5
2. I feel good during my stretches.	1	2	3	4	5

3. I am using positive self-talk before and during the exercise routine.	**1 2 3 4 5**
4. I feel good during my warmup.	**1 2 3 4 5**
5. As I warm up, I plan to give 100% effort.	**1 2 3 4 5**
6. I am determined to complete as much of the exercise session as possible.	**1 2 3 4 5**
7. I try not to think about the stress or strain of exercising.	**1 2 3 4 5**
8. I feel that my exercise performance is improving.	**1 2 3 4 5**
9. I do not think (or care) about what others think of my appearance when I exercise.	**1 2 3 4 5**
10. I try to perform up to my potential.	**1 2 3 4 5**
11. I ignore the appearance, age, gender, and other characteristics of other exercisers.	**1 2 3 4 5**
12. I try to complete as many repetitions as possible of each exercise.	**1 2 3 4 5**
13. I view each exercise bout as a challenge, not a threat.	**1 2 3 4 5**
14. If I feel uncomfortable during exercise, I try to ignore my feelings and focus externally.	**1 2 3 4 5**
15. I remember to try to reach my performance goals.	**1 2 3 4 5**
16. I feel confident in my ability to give 100%.	**1 2 3 4 5**
17. If I get tired, I rest than keep going.	**1 2 3 4 5**

Subtotal: ______

1	2	3	4	5
Not at All Like Me		**Somewhat Like Me**		**Very Much Like Me**

V. After the Exercise Session

1. I am generally pleased with my exercise performance.	1 2 3 4 5
2. I feel that my performance has improved since last time.	1 2 3 4 5
3. I take responsibility for my performance rather than blaming other factors (e.g., poor instructor, noise).	1 2 3 4 5
4. I have recorded (physically or mentally) my progress.	1 2 3 4 5
5. I am open to advice and feedback on my performance.	1 2 3 4 5
6. No matter what level of performance, I plan to keep exercising next time.	1 2 3 4 5
7. I feel good after exercising—a sense of accomplishment.	1 2 3 4 5
8. I reached my target heart rate if I exercised aerobically.	1 2 3 4 5
9. I replace my bodily fluids with water.	1 2 3 4 5
10. My exercise form has improved.	1 2 3 4 5
11. I plan to maintain my exercise program.	1 2 3 4 5

Subtotal ______
GRAND TOTAL: ______

INDEX

Page numbers followed by the letter "t" indicate tables.